THE POWER OF VITAMINS

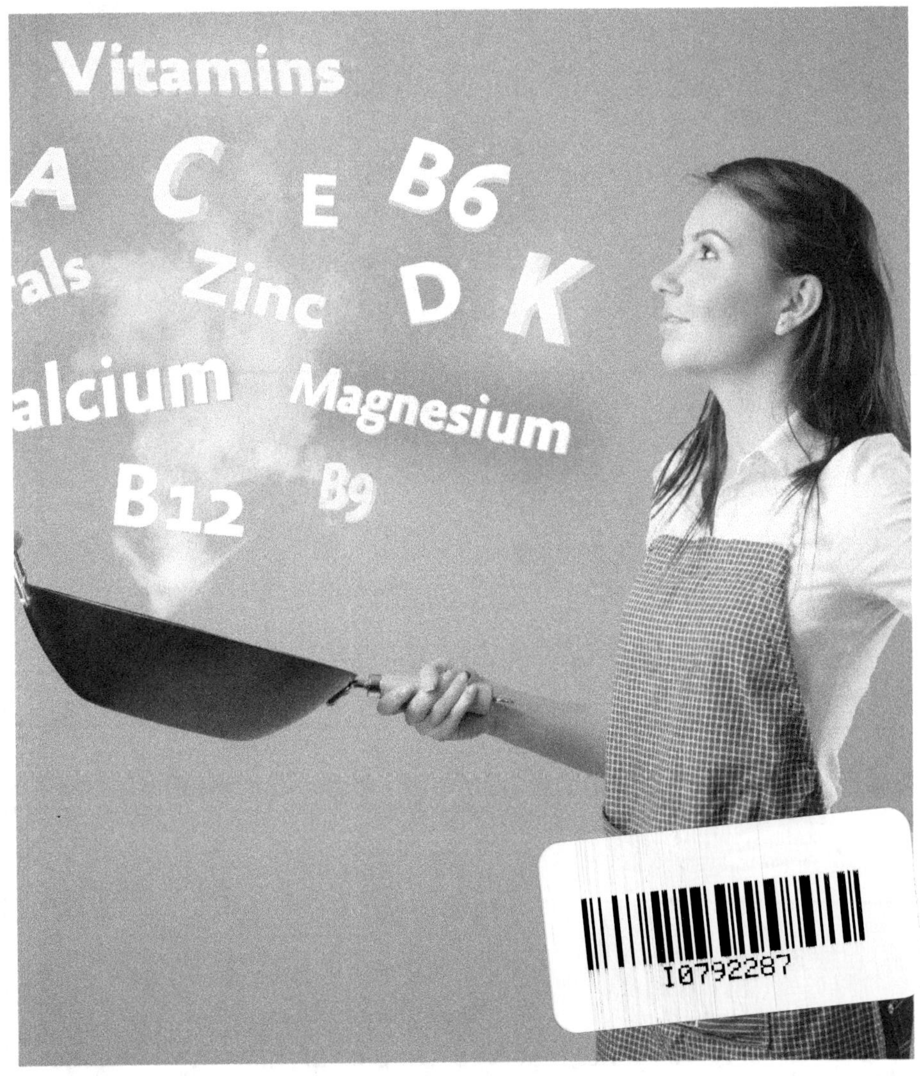

UNDERSTANDING VITAMINS AND THEIR ROLE IN YOUR LIFE

CONTENTS OF THE BOOK:

Chapter 1: The Tale of Tiny Titans – Vitamins and Their Role in Our Lives.. 1

Chapter 2: The Vitamin Chronicles – A Guide to the Alphabet of Health.. 7

Chapter 3: The Vitamin Dilemma – To Supplement or Not?............ 35

Chapter 4: How to Choose the Right Vitamin Supplement – A Practical Guide..40

Chapter 5: Vitamins and Disease Prevention – The Guardians of Long-Term Health...45

Chapter 6: Personalized Vitamin Needs – One Size Doesn't Fit All..51

Chapter 7: Natural Versus Synthetic Vitamins – What's the Difference?.. 55

Chapter 8: Vitamins and Beauty – The Secret to Radiant Skin, Hair, and Nails..61

Conclusion: Embracing the Power of Vitamins.............................. 67

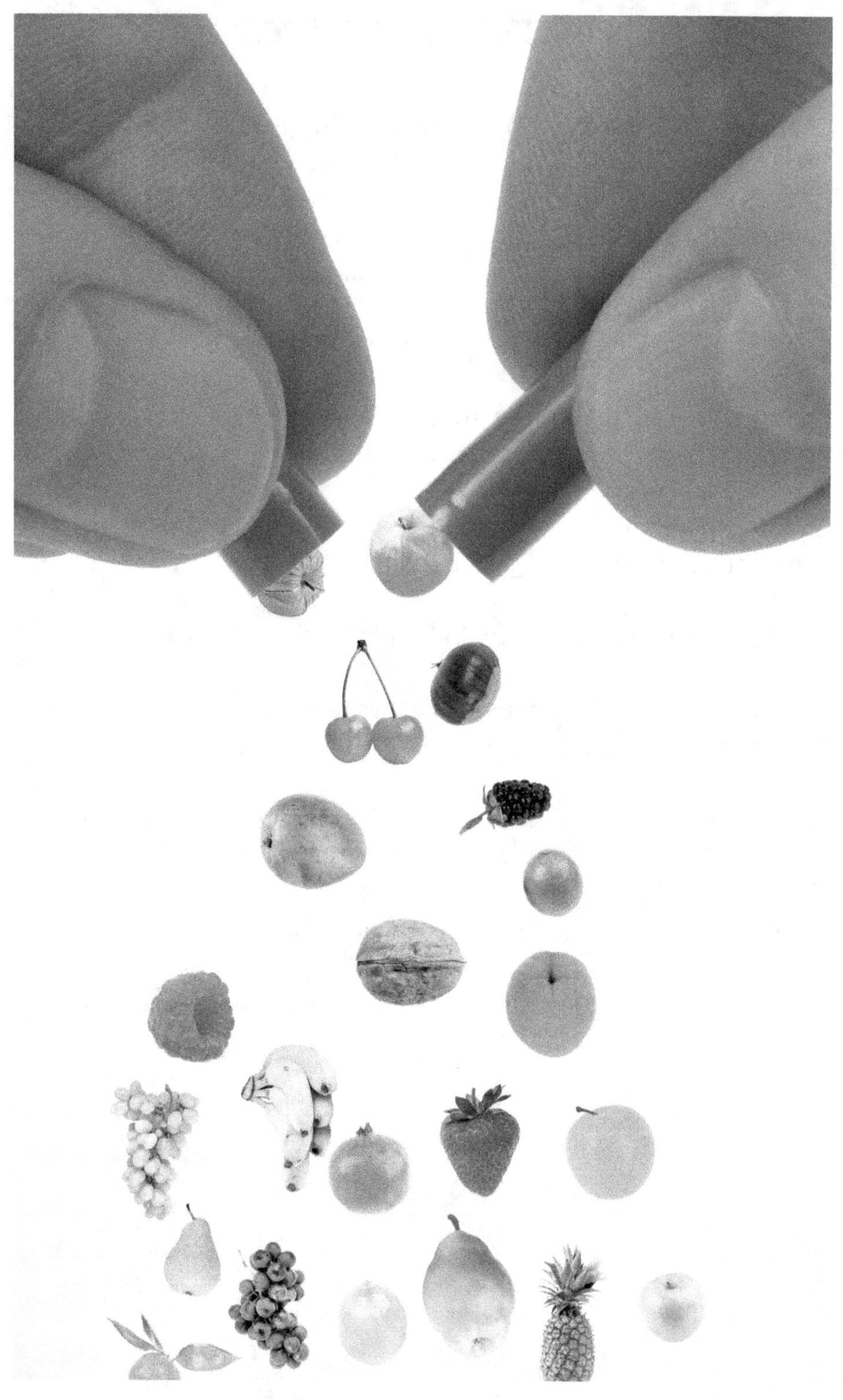

CHAPTER 1:

THE TALE OF TINY TITANS – VITAMINS AND THEIR ROLE IN OUR LIVES

In the vast universe of the human body, there exist tiny, unseen forces that keep everything running smoothly. They don't have the grandeur of the heart pumping life into us or the elegance of our lungs breathing air. Instead, they work silently behind the scenes, ensuring that every cell, tissue, and organ performs its duty. These little heroes are known as vitamins.

The Discovery of Vitamins: A Scientific Adventure

The story of vitamins begins in the late 19th and early 20th centuries—a time when scientists were trying to solve the mysteries of diseases like scurvy, beriberi, and rickets. Unlike infections caused by bacteria or viruses, these illnesses were not contagious. Instead, they seemed to arise from something missing in the diet.

One of the first breakthroughs came when British naval doctor James Lind discovered that sailors who ate citrus fruits like lemons and oranges recovered from scurvy. What Lind didn't know was that these fruits contained a vital substance we now call Vitamin C. This marked the beginning of humanity's understanding of vitamins as essential nutrients.

The term "vitamin" was coined by Polish biochemist Casimir Funk in 1912, derived from "vital amines."

Funk believed these substances were amines (a type of organic compound), though we now know not all vitamins are. The name stuck, and soon the hunt for other vitamins began.

Why Are Vitamins Important?

Imagine your body as a well-designed machine. Each part relies on specific tools and fuels to operate. Vitamins are the tools—small but crucial components that help enzymes perform countless biochemical reactions. Without them, your body's processes would come to a screeching halt.

For example:

✓Vitamin A is the reason you can see in dim light—it helps maintain healthy vision.
✓Vitamin D works with calcium to build strong bones.
✓Vitamin E protects your cells from damage caused by harmful molecules called free radicals.
✓Vitamin K helps your blood clot, preventing excessive bleeding when you get a cut.

Each vitamin has a unique role, and a deficiency can lead to problems that range from mild discomfort to severe health issues.

The Alphabet of Health: Types of Vitamins

Vitamins are divided into two main categories based on how they dissolve in the body:

✦*Fat-Soluble Vitamins (A, D, E, K):*
Stored in the liver and fatty tissues, these vitamins are absorbed along with dietary fat.
They can remain in the body for extended periods, which is why deficiencies are less common but overdoses can be harmful.

✦*Water-Soluble Vitamins (B-complex and C):*
These vitamins dissolve in water and are not stored in the body. They need to be replenished regularly through diet.

B-complex vitamins (like B1, B2, B3, B6, B12, and folic acid) are crucial for energy production and brain function.

Vitamin C is well-known for boosting immunity and repairing tissues.

The Delicate Balance: Benefits and Harms

While vitamins are essential for health, too much of a good thing can be dangerous. Overdosing on fat-soluble vitamins can lead to toxicity.

For instance:

Excessive Vitamin A can cause nausea, dizziness, and even liver damage.

Overloading on Vitamin D can result in calcium buildup in the blood, potentially damaging the heart and kidneys.

This delicate balance is why a well-rounded diet, rather than supplements, is often the best way to meet your vitamin needs.

Signs Your Body Might Be Lacking Vitamins

How do you know if your body is crying out for vitamins? Here are some symptoms that might point to deficiencies:

- Vitamin C deficiency: Bleeding gums, slow-healing wounds, and frequent infections.
- Vitamin D deficiency: Weak bones, fatigue, and muscle pain.
- Vitamin B12 deficiency: Numbness, memory problems, and anemia.
- Vitamin A deficiency: Poor night vision and dry skin.

Each symptom is like a message from your body, urging you to pay attention and provide it with what it needs.

A World of Sources: Where to Find Vitamins

The best way to get your vitamins is through food. Nature offers an incredible variety of sources:

✓Fruits and vegetables are rich in Vitamin C, Vitamin A, and folic acid.

✓Dairy products, fish, and eggs are excellent sources of Vitamin D and B12.

✓Nuts and seeds provide Vitamin E.

✓Leafy greens like spinach and kale are packed with Vitamin K.

A Partnership Between Science and Nature

Today, scientists continue to uncover the roles vitamins play in human health, from preventing chronic diseases to supporting mental well-being. Yet, the most fascinating aspect of vitamins is how they connect us to the natural world. Our reliance on sunlight for Vitamin D, on oranges for Vitamin C, and on leafy greens for Vitamin K is a beautiful reminder of our relationship with the environment.

In Closing: The Vitamin Code

Vitamins are more than just nutrients; they are the secret keepers of health. Understanding them is like cracking a biological code that reveals the incredible machinery of life. So, as you continue reading this book, remember: these tiny titans may be small, but their impact is immeasurable.

In the chapters ahead, we'll dive deeper into the world of vitamins—exploring their specific benefits, sources, and the science behind how they work. Together, we'll uncover the story of life, health, and the incredible role these micronutrients play in it. Let the journey begin!

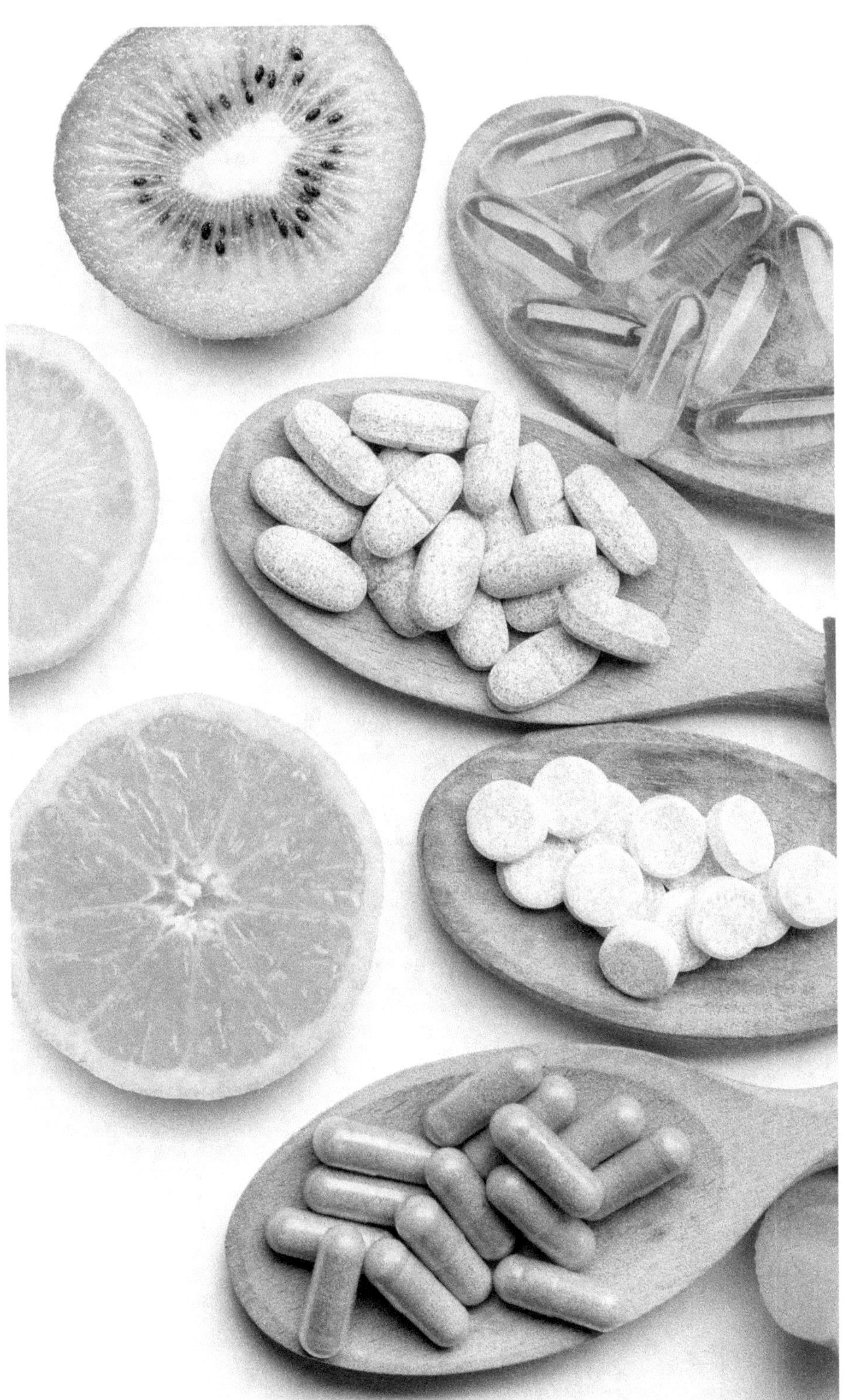

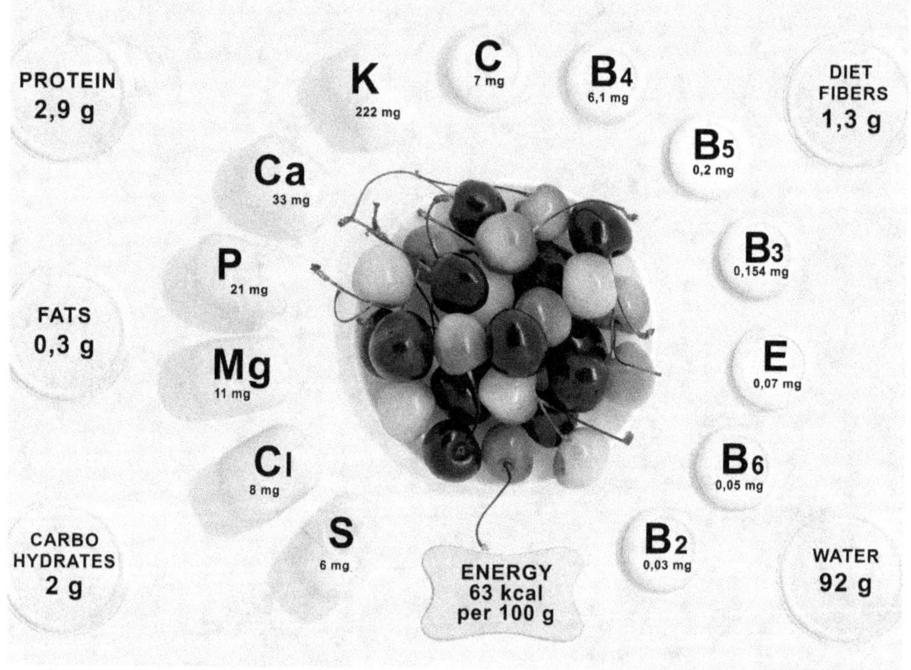

PROTEIN
2,9 g
FATS
0,3 g
CARBO
HYDRATES
2 g
K
222 mg
Ca
33 mg
P
21 mg
Mg
11 mg
Cl
8 mg
S
6 mg
C
7 mg
B_4
6,1 mg
B_5
0,2 mg
B_3
0,154 mg
E
0,07 mg
B_6
0,05 mg
B_2
0,03 mg
ENERGY
63 kcal
per 100 g
DIET
FIBERS
1,3 g
WATER
92 g

CHAPTER 2:

THE VITAMIN CHRONICLES – A GUIDE TO THE ALPHABET OF HEALTH

Now that we've explored the fascinating origins and roles of vitamins, it's time to dive into each one in detail. Each vitamin has its unique characteristics, benefits, and quirks, making them essential pieces of the health puzzle.

VITAMIN A (RETINOL, BETA-CAROTENE)

What It Is and Its Composition

Vitamin A is a fat-soluble vitamin that comes in two primary forms:
- Preformed Vitamin A (Retinol): Found in animal-based foods.
- Provitamin A (Beta-Carotene): Found in plant-based foods, which the body converts into Vitamin A.

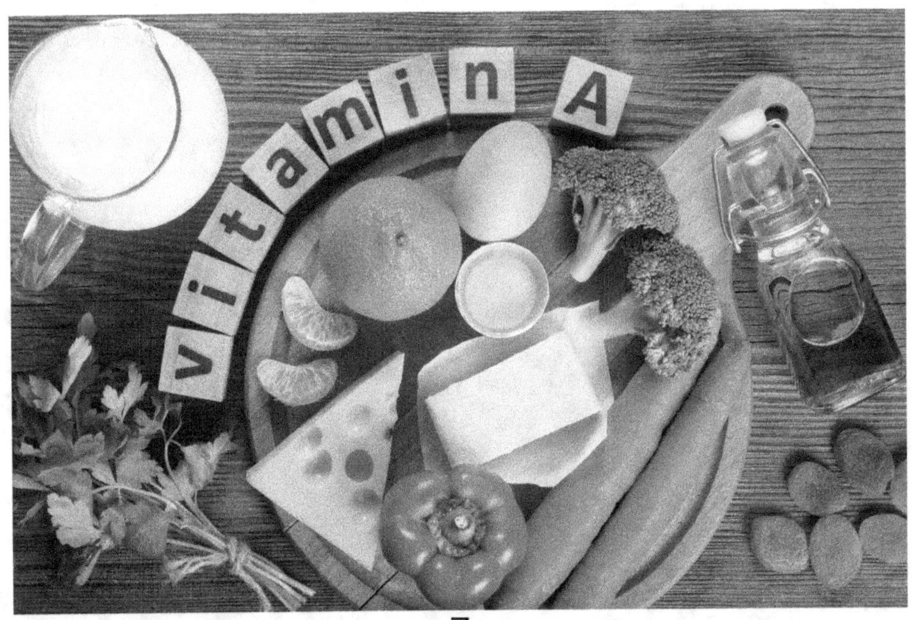

Importance for the Body

Essential for good vision, especially night vision.

Maintains healthy skin and mucous membranes, acting as a barrier to infections.

Supports immune system function.

Plays a role in cell growth and reproduction.

Signs of Deficiency

Night blindness or difficulty seeing in dim light.

Dry, rough skin.

Weakened immune system leading to frequent infections.

Bitot's spots (white patches on the eye).

Benefits

Improves eye health.

Promotes healthy skin and wound healing.

Enhances immunity.

Possible Harms

Overdose can cause toxicity, leading to headaches, dizziness, nausea, and in severe cases, liver damage or birth defects during pregnancy.

Sources

- Animal-based: Liver, fish oil, dairy products, eggs.
- Plant-based: Carrots, sweet potatoes, spinach, and apricots.

VITAMIN B COMPLEX

The Vitamin B group consists of several water-soluble vitamins, each with unique functions:

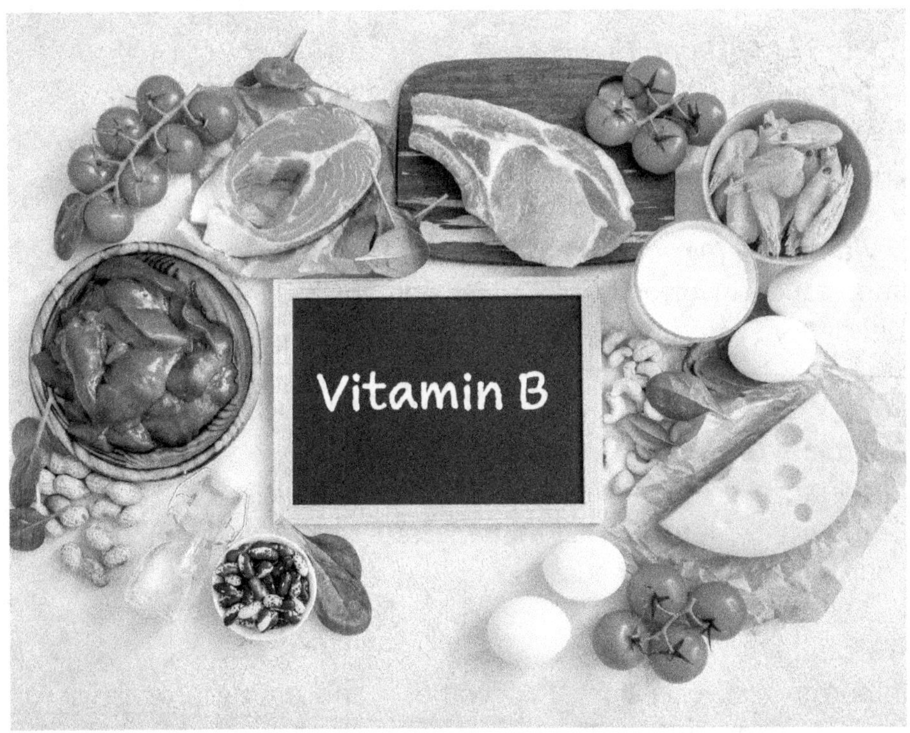

√ *Vitamin B1 (Thiamine)*
Importance: Helps convert food into energy; supports nerve and muscle function.
Deficiency Symptoms: Fatigue, muscle weakness, nerve damage (beriberi).
Sources: Whole grains, pork, legumes.

√ *Vitamin B2 (Riboflavin)*
Importance: Aids in energy production and red blood cell formation.
Deficiency Symptoms: Cracks at the corners of the mouth, sore throat.
Sources: Dairy, almonds, leafy greens.

√ Vitamin B3 (Niacin)

Importance: Supports skin health and nervous system function.
Deficiency Symptoms: Pellagra (diarrhea, dermatitis, dementia).
Sources: Meat, fish, peanuts.

√ Vitamin B5 (Pantothenic Acid)

Importance: Helps produce energy and synthesize hormones.
Deficiency Symptoms: Rare but can cause fatigue and irritability.
Sources: Eggs, avocados, broccoli.

√ Vitamin B6 (Pyridoxine)

Importance: Involved in brain development and immune function.
Deficiency Symptoms: Irritability, depression, weakened immunity.
Sources: Chicken, bananas, potatoes.

√ Vitamin B7 (Biotin)

Importance: Promotes healthy hair, skin, and nails.
Deficiency Symptoms: Hair thinning, skin rashes.
Sources: Eggs, nuts, seeds.

√ Vitamin B9 (Folic Acid)

Importance: Crucial for DNA synthesis and during pregnancy for fetal development.
Deficiency Symptoms: Anemia, birth defects.
Sources: Leafy greens, citrus fruits, fortified cereals.

√ Vitamin B12 (Cobalamin)

Importance: Necessary for red blood cell production and nerve function.
Deficiency Symptoms: Fatigue, numbness, memory issues.
Sources: Meat, fish, dairy (vegans may need supplements).

VITAMIN C (ASCORBIC ACID)

What It Is and Its Composition

Vitamin C is a water-soluble vitamin composed of carbon, hydrogen, and oxygen molecules.

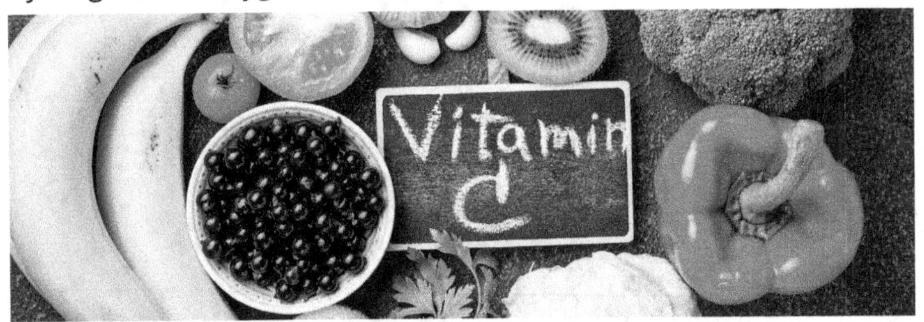

Importance for the Body

Boosts the immune system.
Aids in collagen production, essential for skin, bones, and connective tissue.
Acts as a powerful antioxidant.

Signs of Deficiency

Scurvy (bleeding gums, fatigue, joint pain).
Frequent infections.
Slow wound healing.

Benefits

Improves skin elasticity.
Enhances iron absorption from plant-based foods.
Reduces the risk of chronic diseases.

Possible Harms

Overconsumption can cause digestive discomfort, including diarrhea and nausea.

Sources

Citrus fruits (oranges, lemons), strawberries, bell peppers, and broccoli.

<u>*VITAMIN D (CALCIFEROL)*</u>

What It Is and Its Composition

Vitamin D is a fat-soluble vitamin synthesized in the skin when exposed to sunlight.

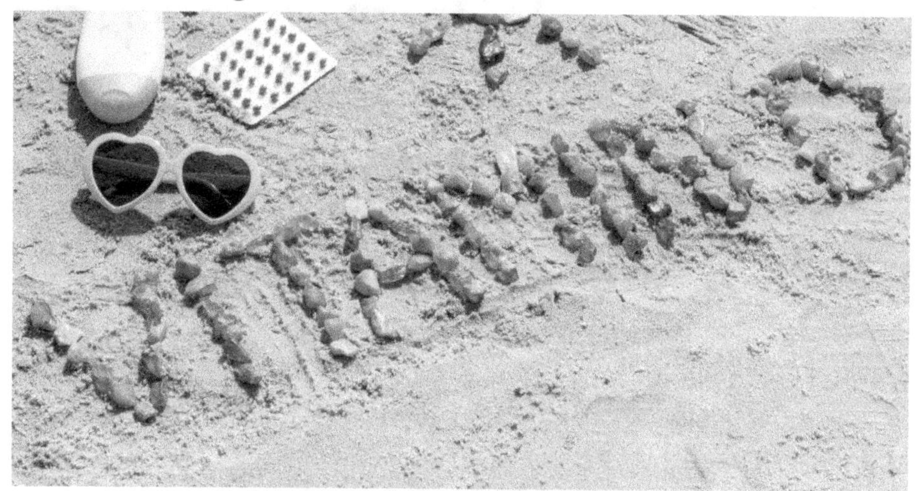

Importance for the Body

Enhances calcium absorption, crucial for strong bones and teeth.
Supports muscle and immune function.

Signs of Deficiency

Rickets in children (soft, weak bones).
Osteomalacia in adults (bone pain, muscle weakness).
Increased susceptibility to infections.

Benefits

Prevents bone disorders like osteoporosis.
May boost mood and reduce depression symptoms.

Possible Harms

Excess can cause hypercalcemia (high calcium levels), leading to kidney damage.

Sources

Sunlight exposure, fatty fish, fortified dairy products.

VITAMIN E (TOCOPHEROL)

What It Is and Its Composition

A fat-soluble antioxidant that protects cells from free radical damage.

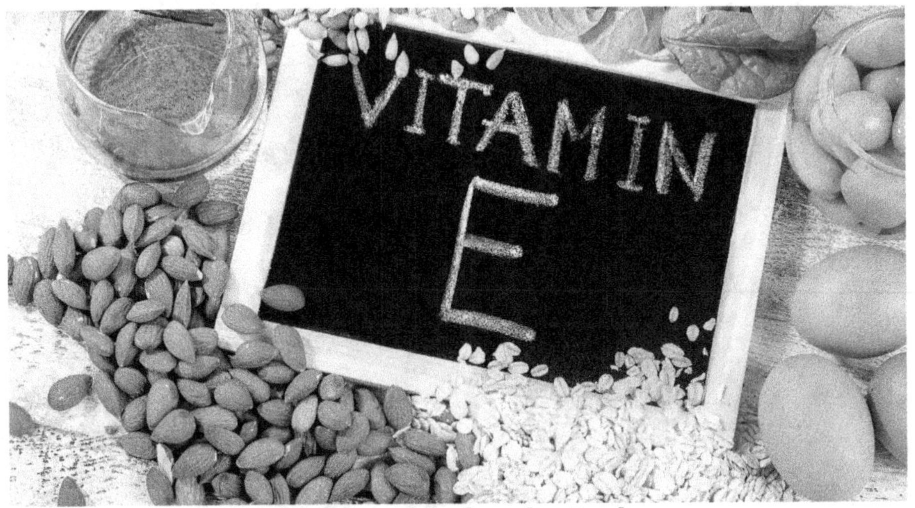

Importance for the Body

Maintains healthy skin and eyes.
Strengthens the immune system.

Signs of Deficiency

Rare but can include nerve and muscle damage, vision problems.

Benefits

Supports skin health.
Protects against chronic diseases caused by oxidative stress.

Possible Harms

Excessive intake can interfere with blood clotting and lead to hemorrhage.

Sources

Nuts, seeds, vegetable oils, spinach.

<u>***VITAMIN K***</u>

What It Is and Its Composition

A fat-soluble vitamin essential for blood clotting and bone metabolism.

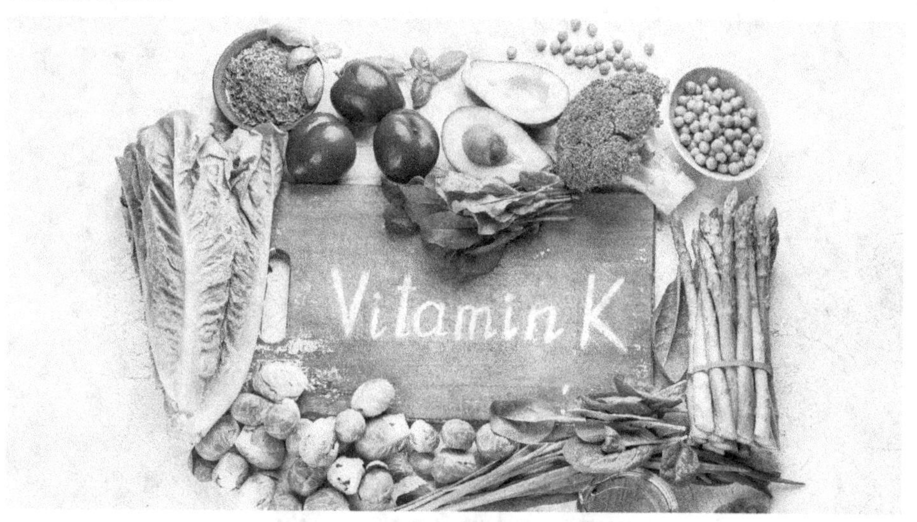

Importance for the Body
Prevents excessive bleeding by aiding blood clotting.
Supports bone strength.

Signs of Deficiency
Easy bruising and excessive bleeding.
Bone fractures.

Benefits
Promotes faster wound healing.
Reduces risk of osteoporosis.

Possible Harms
No known toxic effects, but those on blood thinners should monitor intake.

Sources
Leafy greens, broccoli, and fermented foods.

<u>*CHOLINE*</u>

What It Is and Its Composition

Choline is a water-soluble compound, often grouped with the B-complex vitamins, though it is not officially classified as a vitamin. It contains nitrogen and is essential for synthesizing acetylcholine, a key neurotransmitter.

Importance for the Body
Supports brain development and function.
Aids in the formation of cell membranes.
Helps metabolize fats in the liver.

Signs of Deficiency
Fatty liver disease (hepatic steatosis).
Memory issues or cognitive decline.
Muscle damage.

Benefits
Promotes brain health and may reduce the risk of neurological disorders.
Improves liver health by preventing fat buildup.

Possible Harms
Excessive intake can cause fishy body odor, low blood pressure, and sweating.

Sources
Eggs, liver, fish, nuts, broccoli, and cauliflower.

INOSITOL

What It Is and Its Composition

Inositol, sometimes referred to as Vitamin B8, is a sugar-like compound found naturally in cells. Though not officially a vitamin, it has vitamin-like properties.

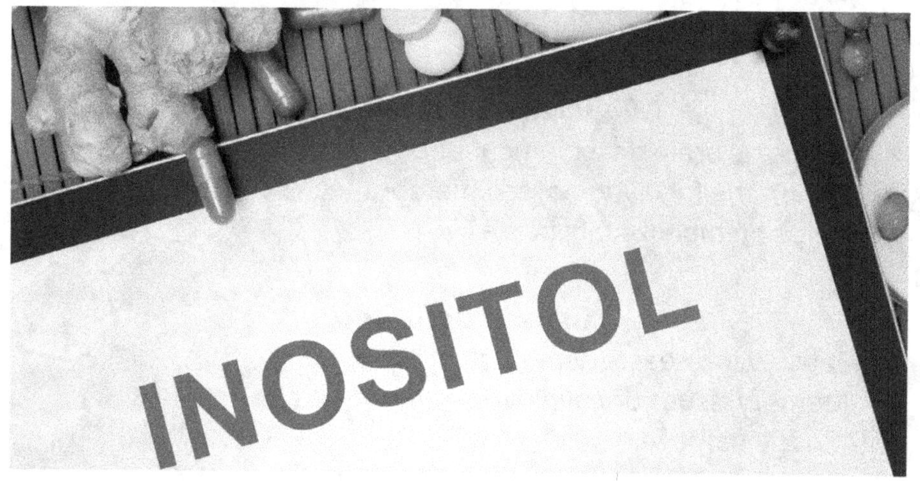

Importance for the Body

Plays a role in cell signaling and the functioning of insulin. Important for mental health and mood regulation.

Signs of Deficiency

Rare in healthy individuals, but low levels may affect insulin sensitivity or mental health.

Benefits

May reduce symptoms of anxiety and depression.
Supports reproductive health by improving ovarian function in conditions like PCOS (Polycystic Ovary Syndrome).

Possible Harms

Generally safe, but high doses can cause digestive discomfort.

Sources

Citrus fruits, beans, nuts, whole grains.

VITAMIN F (ESSENTIAL FATTY ACIDS)

What It Is and Its Composition

Vitamin F refers to essential fatty acids, primarily Omega-3 and Omega-6, which are vital fats that the body cannot produce on its own.

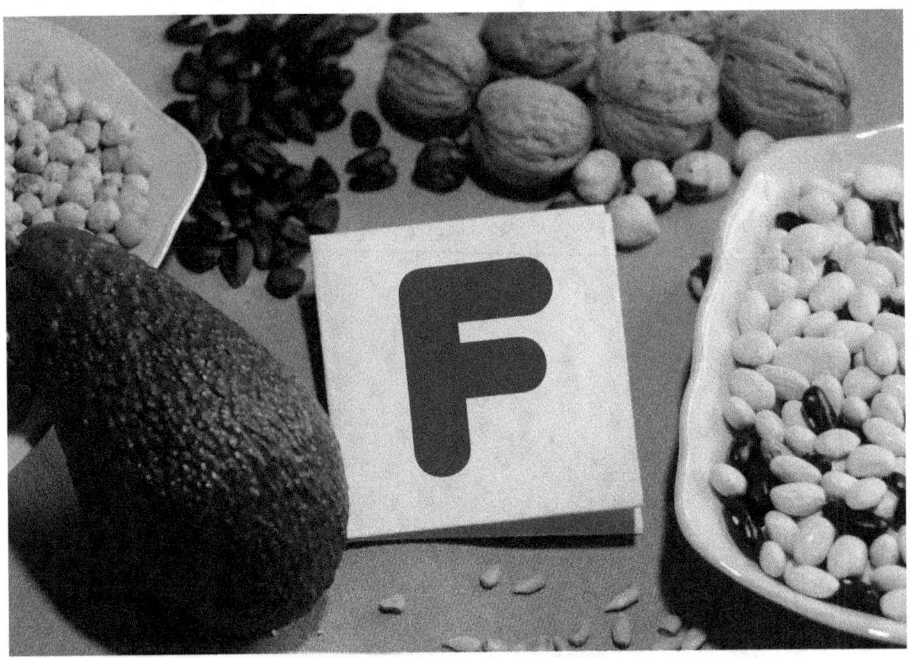

Importance for the Body

Vital for brain health and development.
Reduces inflammation and supports heart health.

Signs of Deficiency

Dry, scaly skin.
Hair loss.
Poor wound healing.

Benefits

Improves cardiovascular health by reducing cholesterol levels.
Enhances skin and hair health.
Supports mental health by improving mood and cognitive

function.

Possible Harms
Excess Omega-6, without balancing Omega-3, may contribute to inflammation.

Sources
- Omega-3: Fatty fish (salmon, mackerel), walnuts, flaxseeds.
- Omega-6: Vegetable oils (sunflower, soybean), nuts, seeds.

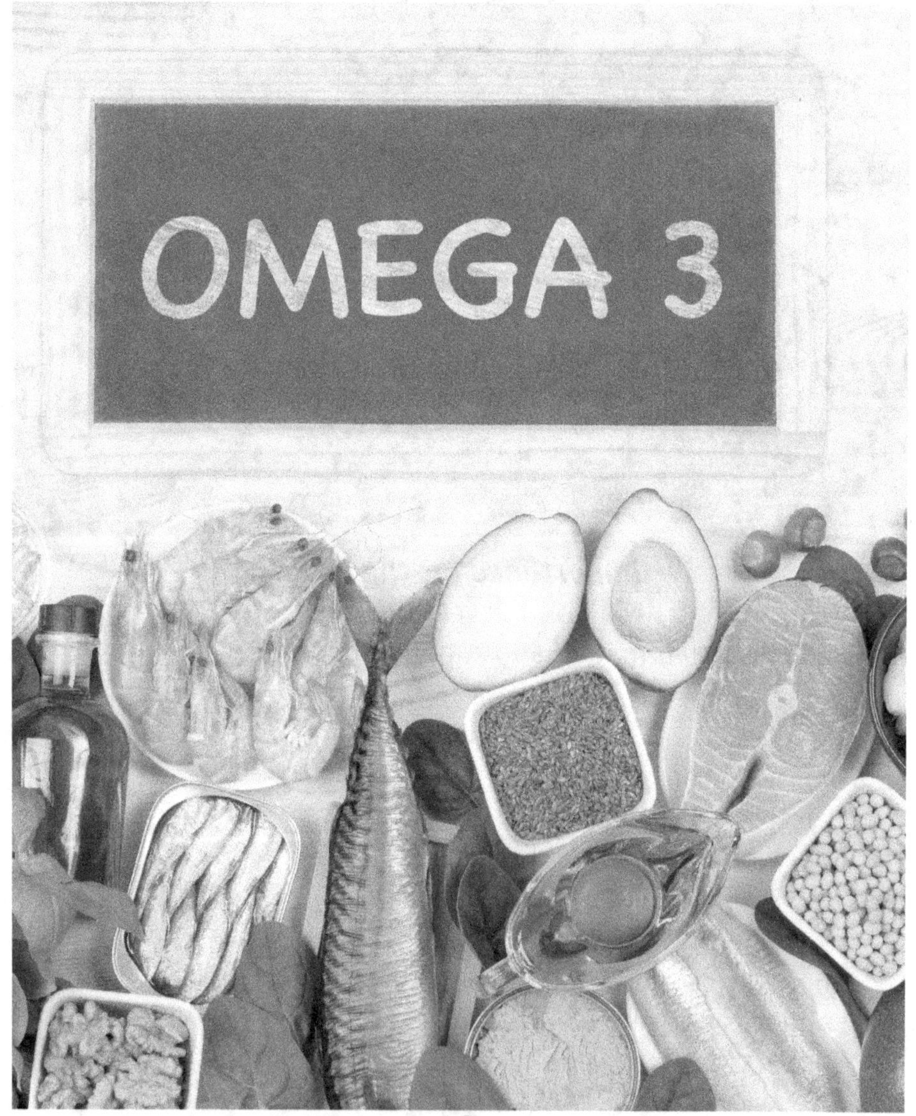

CALCIUM

What It Is

Calcium is a mineral essential for building and maintaining strong bones and teeth. It also plays a critical role in muscle function, nerve signaling, and blood clotting.

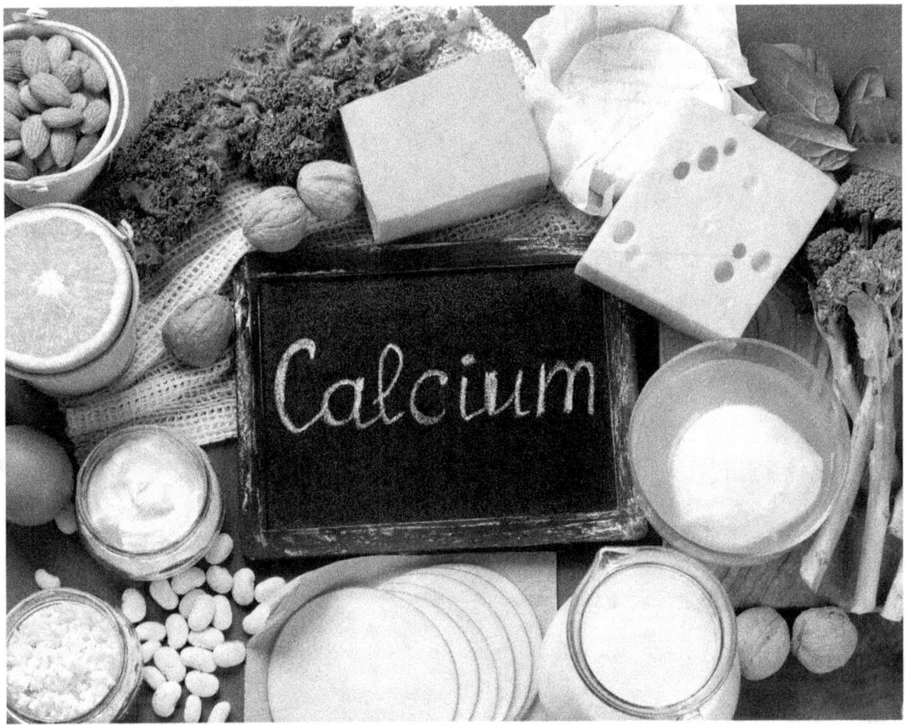

Importance for the Body

Strengthens bones and teeth.
Supports muscle contractions and relaxation.
Assists in nerve transmission and communication.
Aids in blood clot formation.

Signs of Deficiency

Weak or brittle bones (osteoporosis).
Muscle cramps or spasms.
Numbness or tingling in fingers.
Increased risk of fractures.

Benefits

Reduces the risk of osteoporosis and bone-related diseases.
Helps maintain a steady heartbeat.
Supports proper hormonal secretion.

Possible Harms

Excess calcium (hypercalcemia) can lead to kidney stones, constipation, or calcium deposits in soft tissues.

High doses may interfere with the absorption of other minerals, such as iron and zinc.

Sources

- Dairy products: Milk, cheese, yogurt.
- Leafy greens: Kale, spinach, broccoli.
- Fortified foods: Orange juice, plant-based milk, cereals.
- Fish: Sardines, salmon (with bones).

MAGNESIUM

What It Is

Magnesium is a vital mineral involved in over 300 biochemical reactions in the body. It is essential for energy production, muscle function, and maintaining a healthy nervous system.

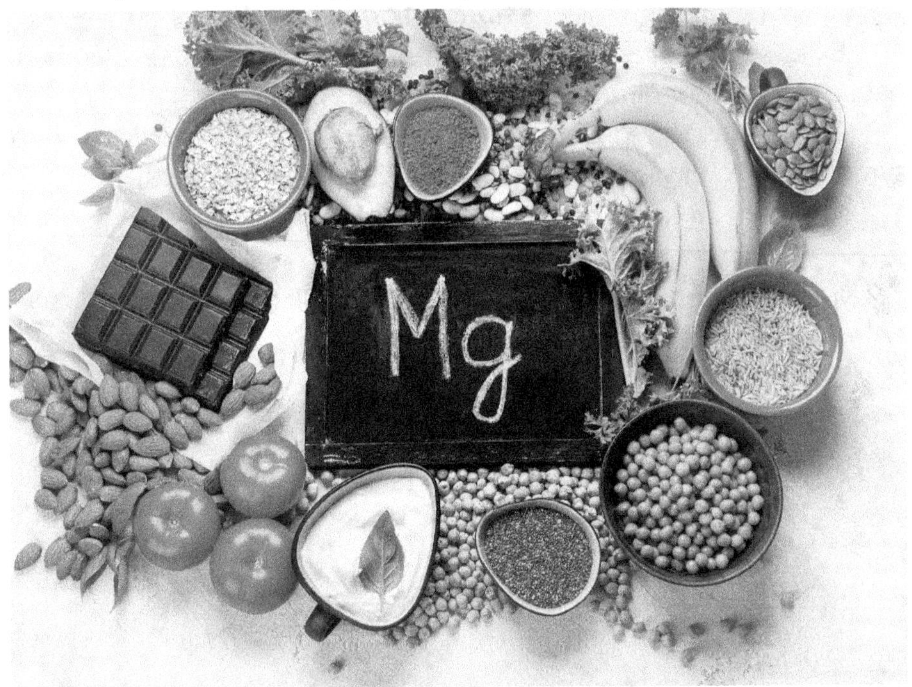

Importance for the Body

Regulates muscle and nerve function.
Supports the synthesis of DNA and proteins.
Helps convert food into energy.
Maintains healthy blood pressure and heartbeat rhythm.

Signs of Deficiency

Muscle twitches, cramps, or spasms.
Fatigue or weakness.
Irregular heartbeat.
Increased risk of migraines or anxiety.

Benefits

Promotes relaxation and reduces stress.

Helps prevent migraines and muscle cramps.

Enhances bone health by working alongside calcium and Vitamin D.

Supports healthy blood sugar levels.

Possible Harms

Excessive magnesium from supplements can cause diarrhea, nausea, and abdominal cramps.

Extremely high doses may lead to magnesium toxicity, with symptoms like low blood pressure and irregular heartbeat.

Sources

- Nuts and seeds: Almonds, cashews, pumpkin seeds.
- Whole grains: Brown rice, quinoa, oats.
- Leafy greens: Spinach, Swiss chard.
- Legumes: Black beans, lentils.
- Seafood: Salmon, mackerel.

VITAMIN P (BIOFLAVONOIDS)

What It Is and Its Composition

Vitamin P is a group of plant compounds, known as flavonoids, that are not true vitamins but have vitamin-like effects.

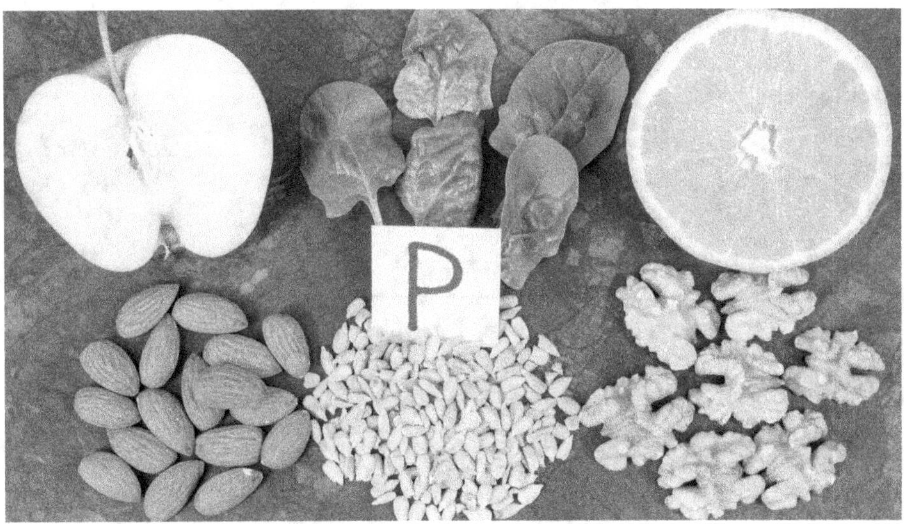

Importance for the Body

Enhances the absorption of Vitamin C.
Strengthens blood vessel walls.
Acts as an antioxidant.

Signs of Deficiency

Rare, but weak capillaries can lead to easy bruising or bleeding gums.

Benefits

Protects against heart disease by improving blood circulation.
Reduces inflammation and fights oxidative stress.

Possible Harms

Generally safe; no known toxic effects.

Sources

Citrus fruits, berries, green tea, dark chocolate.

CARNITINE

What It Is and Its Composition

Carnitine is a nutrient that helps transport fatty acids into the mitochondria, where they are converted into energy. Like choline, it is not officially classified as a vitamin but is crucial for energy metabolism.

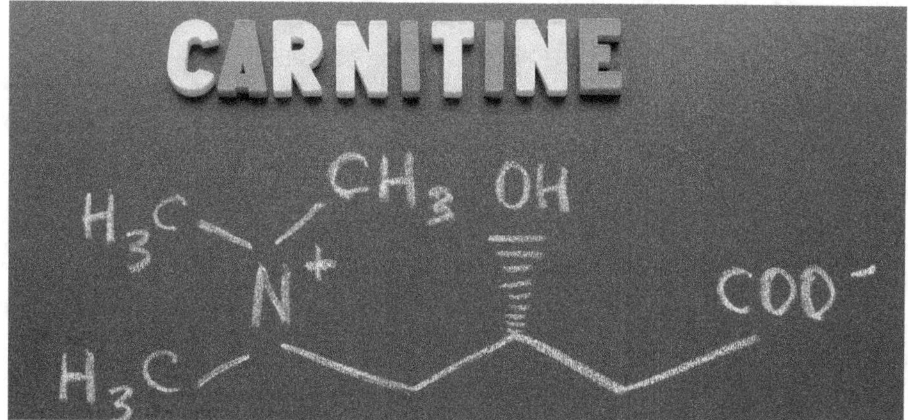

Importance for the Body

Essential for energy production, particularly during exercise. Supports heart and brain health.

Signs of Deficiency

Fatigue and muscle weakness.
Heart or liver issues in severe cases.

Benefits

Boosts athletic performance and endurance.
May improve symptoms of certain conditions, like heart disease and diabetic neuropathy.

Possible Harms

High doses can cause nausea, vomiting, or a "fishy" body odor.

Sources

Meat, fish, poultry, milk, and whole grains.

COENZYME Q10 (COQ10)

What It Is and Its Composition

Coenzyme Q10 is a fat-soluble compound found in all cells. It plays a key role in energy production and functions as a powerful antioxidant.

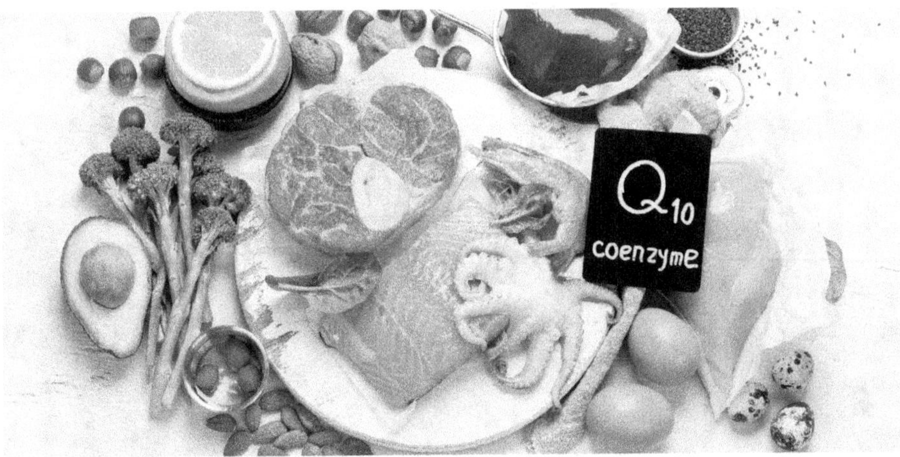

Importance for the Body

Supports energy production in cells.
Protects cells from oxidative damage.

Signs of Deficiency

Fatigue and weakness.
Heart or muscle-related symptoms.

Benefits

Improves energy levels, particularly in individuals with chronic fatigue.
Supports heart health and may reduce blood pressure.

Possible Harms

Generally safe, but high doses can cause digestive upset.

Sources

Fatty fish, organ meats, nuts, seeds.

<u>LIPOIC ACID (ALPHA-LIPOIC ACID)</u>

What It Is and Its Composition

Lipoic acid is a vitamin-like compound that helps enzymes convert nutrients into energy.

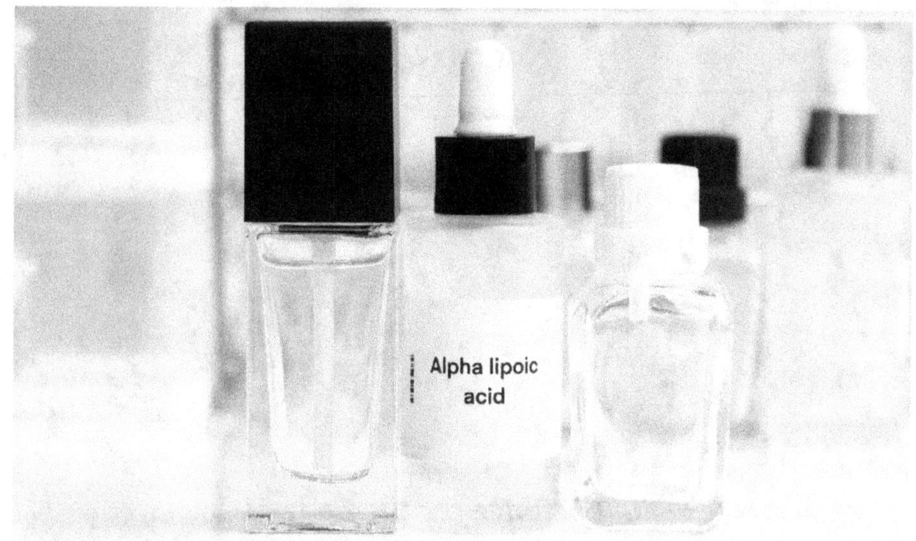

Importance for the Body
Acts as a potent antioxidant.
Helps regenerate other antioxidants, like Vitamin C and E.

Signs of Deficiency
Rare, but may include fatigue or impaired glucose metabolism.

Benefits
Helps control blood sugar levels.
May reduce symptoms of nerve pain (neuropathy).

Possible Harms
High doses can cause nausea or skin rashes.

Sources
Spinach, broccoli, potatoes, organ meats.

PABA (PARA-AMINOBENZOIC ACID)

What It Is and Its Composition

PABA is often considered part of the B-complex group, though it is not a true vitamin. It is a component of folic acid and supports many biochemical processes.

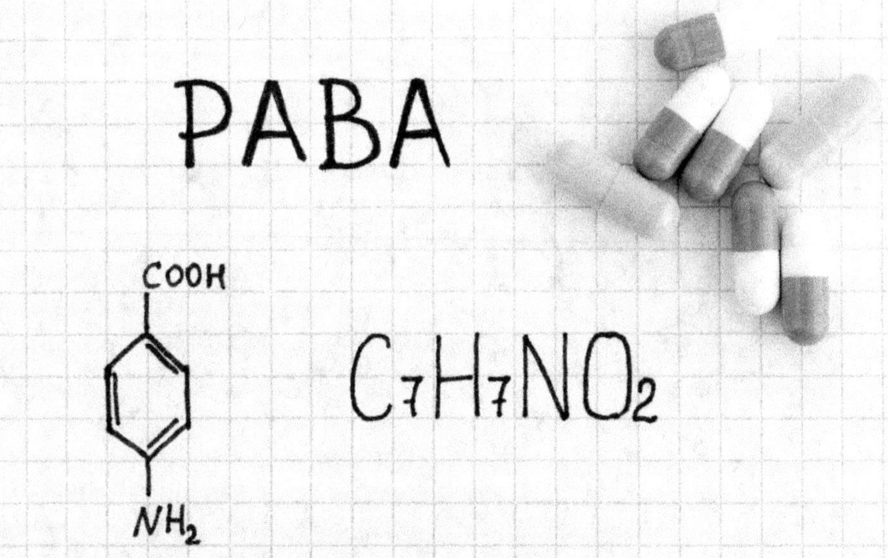

Importance for the Body
Assists in the synthesis of folic acid in the body.
May promote healthy skin and hair pigmentation.

Signs of Deficiency
Rare, as it is produced by gut bacteria.
Premature graying of hair and potential skin conditions have been linked to insufficient levels.

Benefits
May protect skin from UV damage (it is used in sunscreens).
Potential to improve skin conditions like eczema.

Possible Harms
Overdose can cause nausea, vomiting, and liver damage in rare

cases.

Liver, eggs, molasses, whole grains.

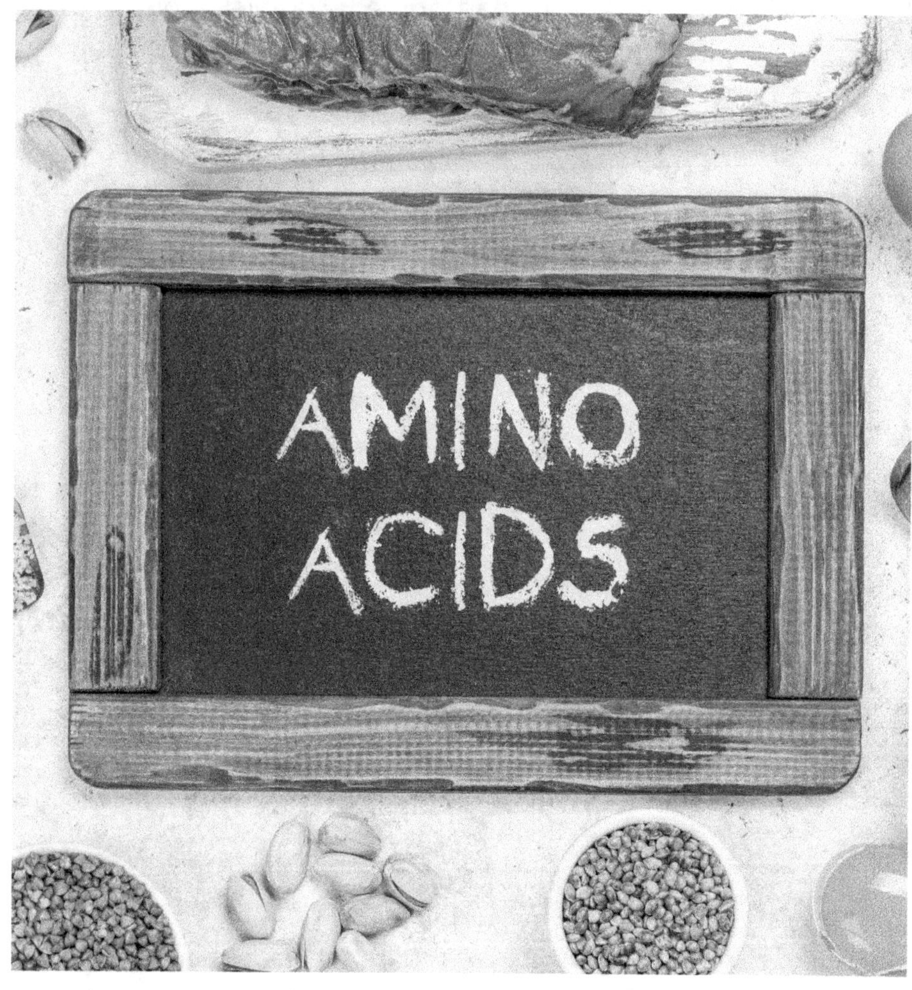

What It Is and Its Composition

Taurine, sometimes referred to as Vitamin T, is an amino acid-like compound rather than a true vitamin. It is vital for several physiological processes.

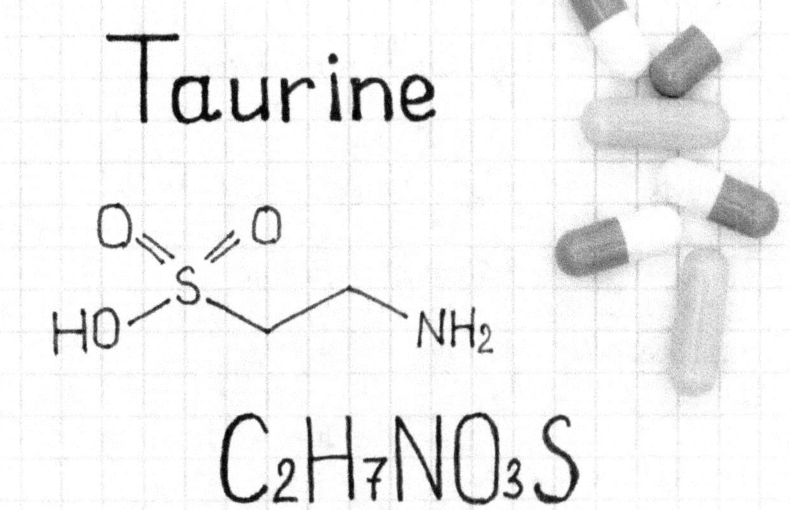

Importance for the Body
Crucial for brain and heart function.
Supports muscle development and bile salt production.

Signs of Deficiency
Rare, but symptoms may include fatigue, muscle weakness, or impaired vision.

Benefits
Improves athletic performance and endurance.
Supports eye and cardiovascular health.

Possible Harms
High intake may cause slight digestive upset.

Sources
Found naturally in meat, fish, and dairy products.

VITAMIN H2 (MENATETRENONE)

What It Is and Its Composition

Vitamin H2 is another form of Vitamin K2, known as menaquinone-4 (MK-4), and is important for calcium regulation in the body.

Importance for the Body

Directs calcium to bones and teeth, preventing buildup in arteries.

Works alongside Vitamin D to enhance bone health.

Signs of Deficiency

Weak bones or increased risk of fractures.
Calcification of blood vessels.

Benefits

Reduces the risk of osteoporosis.
Supports cardiovascular health.

Possible Harms

No known toxicity at normal dietary levels.

Sources

Meat, eggs, and fermented foods like natto.

VITAMIN PQQ (PYRROLOQUINOLINE QUINONE)

What It Is and Its Composition

PQQ is a newly discovered compound with vitamin-like qualities, important for cellular growth and mitochondrial function.

Importance for the Body
Supports the production of new mitochondria.
Enhances brain function and cognitive health.

Signs of Deficiency
Still under research, but low levels may affect brain and energy function.

Benefits
Improves cognitive performance.
May reduce the effects of aging by supporting cellular health.

Possible Harms
Excessive doses may cause mild digestive upset.

Sources
- Kiwi, papaya, green tea, and fermented soy products.
- Ortho-Molecular Vitamins (Hypothetical Compounds)
- Ortho-molecular vitamins represent an advanced concept in nutritional science. These are compounds theorized to act as "designer vitamins," tailored to enhance the biochemical individuality of humans.

<u>***VITAMIN N (LIPOIC ACID)***</u>

What It Is and Its Composition

Vitamin N, another term for Alpha-Lipoic Acid (covered earlier), deserves emphasis for its dual nature as both a fat- and water-soluble antioxidant.

Importance for the Body
Regenerates other antioxidants like Vitamins C and E.
Improves nerve health.

Signs of Deficiency
Rare, but could include fatigue or neuropathy.

Benefits
Protects against oxidative stress and diabetes-related nerve damage.

Possible Harms
Excessive amounts may cause a drop in blood sugar levels.

Sources
Red meat, organ meats, and vegetables like spinach.

<u>*VITAMIN U (S-METHYLMETHIONINE)*</u>

What It Is and Its Composition

Vitamin U is a compound found in cabbage and other cruciferous vegetables. Though not a true vitamin, it has protective effects on the digestive system.

Importance for the Body

Helps heal the lining of the stomach and intestines.
Reduces the risk of ulcers.

Signs of Deficiency

Not typically discussed, as it's not classified as essential.

Benefits

Supports gut health.
May aid in digestion and reduce inflammation.

Possible Harms

No known toxic effects.

Sources

Cabbage, broccoli, Brussels sprouts.

Conclusion

Each vitamin is a unique piece of the health puzzle, indispensable for maintaining balance in the body. Understanding their roles, benefits, and potential harms empowers us to make better dietary and lifestyle choices. The key to unlocking the full potential of these micronutrients lies in balance, moderation, and an appreciation for the diverse foods that provide them.

The world of vitamins extends beyond the familiar A through K. These additional compounds like choline, inositol, and CoQ10 illustrate the intricate biochemistry that sustains life. While they may not all be classified as "vitamins," their roles are no less important in maintaining optimal health.

CHAPTER 3:

THE VITAMIN DILEMMA – TO SUPPLEMENT OR NOT?

In an age of health-conscious living, the shelves of pharmacies and grocery stores are stocked with rows upon rows of vitamin supplements promising vitality, longevity, and enhanced well-being. While the allure of these promises can be strong, the question remains: Should we take vitamins on our own without medical guidance?

This chapter dives into the potential benefits, risks, and considerations of self-supplementing vitamins, aiming to shed light on a complex and important topic.

The Temptation of Self-Supplementation

Vitamin supplements are marketed as convenient, easy solutions to bridge the gap between our diets and our body's needs.

The appeal is undeniable:

- A pill promises to correct deficiencies and boost health.
- Busy lifestyles often leave little time to prepare nutrient-rich meals.
- Online health advice and anecdotal stories make supplements seem universally beneficial.

However, is self-supplementing always a good idea? Let's explore the nuances.

The Body's Complex Needs

Each individual has unique nutritional requirements based on factors like age, gender, activity level, health conditions, and even genetics. While supplements can help in specific cases, the body generally prefers to receive nutrients from whole foods. Here's why:

✓Bioavailability: Vitamins in food are often more easily absorbed because they come with complementary nutrients, like fiber, fats, and minerals.

✓Synergistic Effects: Whole foods provide a balance of nutrients that work together, such as Vitamin C enhancing iron absorption.

✓Safety Mechanisms: Foods naturally limit excessive nutrient intake, whereas supplements can easily lead to overdosing.

By self-supplementing without understanding your body's specific needs, you may upset these delicate balances.

The Risks of Excessive Vitamin Use

Many people mistakenly believe that "more is better" when it comes to vitamins. However, taking high doses of certain vitamins can cause serious health issues. These risks vary depending on the vitamin:

◆*Fat-Soluble Vitamins (A, D, E, K): The Culprits of Toxicity*
These vitamins are stored in the liver and fatty tissues, meaning the body does not easily excrete them.

Overconsumption can lead to:

◆*Vitamin A toxicity (Hypervitaminosis A):* Symptoms include nausea, dizziness, headaches, and in severe cases, liver damage or birth defects during pregnancy.

◆*Vitamin D toxicity (Hypercalcemia):* Excess calcium in the blood can cause kidney damage, irregular heartbeats, and confusion.

◆*Vitamin E overdose:* Interferes with blood clotting, increasing the risk of bleeding.

◆*Vitamin K overdose:* Rare, but excessive amounts may counteract blood-thinning medications.

Water-Soluble Vitamins (B-complex, C): The False Sense of Safety

These vitamins are less likely to cause toxicity because excess amounts are excreted in urine. However, mega-doses can still lead to problems:

- Vitamin C: Overuse may cause kidney stones, diarrhea, and nausea.
- Vitamin B6: High doses over time can lead to nerve damage, causing numbness or tingling.

Interactions with Medications

Certain vitamins can interact negatively with medications:

- Vitamin K may reduce the effectiveness of blood thinners like warfarin.
- Vitamin E and fish oil supplements can increase bleeding risk when combined with anticoagulants.
- High doses of Vitamin C can interfere with chemotherapy drugs.

The Psychological Aspect: The Placebo Effect

Interestingly, some benefits people attribute to self-supplementation might stem from the placebo effect. When people take vitamins, they often believe they are healthier, which can lead to positive behavioral changes, like exercising more or eating better. These changes, rather than the supplements themselves, may drive improved health.

When Are Supplements Necessary?

While self-supplementation can be risky, there are legitimate scenarios where supplements are beneficial or necessary:

✓Vitamin D Deficiency: For those with limited sun exposure, such as individuals living in northern climates, Vitamin D supplements are often recommended.

✔Pregnancy: Folate (Vitamin B9) is critical for preventing neural tube defects in the developing fetus.

✔Vegan or Vegetarian Diets: Vitamin B12 is almost exclusively found in animal products, making supplementation essential for those avoiding meat.

✔Age-Related Needs: Older adults may require calcium, Vitamin D, or Vitamin B12 due to reduced absorption.

✔Medical Conditions: Certain illnesses or surgeries, such as gastric bypass, can impair nutrient absorption.

In such cases, supplementation should be done under medical supervision to ensure appropriate dosages.

Guidelines for Safe Vitamin Use

If you decide to take vitamins, here are some general rules to follow:

◆Consult a Healthcare Professional: A doctor can recommend specific supplements based on blood tests and your medical history.

◆Start with Food: Prioritize getting vitamins from nutrient-dense foods.

For example:

- Spinach, kale, and carrots for Vitamin A.
- Citrus fruits and bell peppers for Vitamin C.
- Fatty fish, eggs, and fortified foods for Vitamin D.

◆Avoid Mega-Doses: Stick to the recommended daily allowance (RDA) unless advised otherwise.

◆Read Labels Carefully: Some multivitamins provide doses far exceeding the RDA, which can be harmful over time.

◆Be Cautious of Fad Supplements: Beware of supplements claiming to "boost energy" or "detoxify the body"—many are unregulated and lack scientific backing.

The Role of Medical Supervision

Doctors and dietitians have access to diagnostic tools like

blood tests that can reveal deficiencies or excesses. They can also monitor your progress to adjust dosages if needed. Attempting to self-diagnose nutrient needs risks creating new problems or worsening existing ones.

A Balanced Perspective

It's important to recognize that vitamins are not magical cures for all ailments. They are essential micronutrients that support overall health, but their benefits are maximized when:

- They are part of a balanced diet.
- They are taken under medical advice when necessary.
- Lifestyle factors like exercise, sleep, and stress management are also addressed.

Conclusion: A Thoughtful Approach

The decision to take vitamins should not be made lightly. While they can offer tremendous health benefits, they also carry risks when used improperly. The best strategy is to listen to your body, rely on whole foods, and seek professional guidance when supplements are required.

In the next chapter, we'll explore how to assess vitamin quality, decipher supplement labels, and ensure you're making the best choices for your health. The journey to understanding vitamins continues!

CHAPTER 4:

HOW TO CHOOSE THE RIGHT VITAMIN SUPPLEMENT – A PRACTICAL GUIDE

The supplement market can feel overwhelming, with countless options promising better health, more energy, and disease prevention. Choosing the right vitamin supplement requires careful attention to labels, certifications, and sourcing.

This chapter serves as your step-by-step guide to making informed decisions, avoiding low-quality products, and understanding the key terms used in supplement labeling.

1. Decoding Supplement Labels

The supplement facts label provides vital information about the product. Understanding its components is the first step in making an informed choice.

Key Terms to Know

- RDA (Recommended Dietary Allowance): The daily intake level of a nutrient sufficient to meet the needs of most healthy individuals. Supplements often aim to meet or exceed the RDA.
- DV (Daily Value): A percentage indicating how much of a nutrient the supplement provides relative to general dietary recommendations for a 2,000-calorie diet.

Example: If a label says 50% DV for Vitamin C, one serving provides half the daily recommended intake.

- IU (International Units): A measurement used for vitamins like A, D, and E to express potency based on biological activity rather than weight.

Example: 1 IU of Vitamin D equals 0.025 micrograms of cholecalciferol.

- MCG/ MG (Micrograms/ Milligrams): The weight of a nutrient in the supplement. (1,000 mcg = 1 mg).

40

Common Sections on a Label
- Serving Size: Indicates the number of pills, capsules, or drops required for one dose.
- Amount Per Serving: The quantity of each nutrient provided in a single serving.
- Ingredients List: Details all active and inactive ingredients, including fillers, binders, or flavorings.
- Other Ingredients: Additional compounds, such as gelatin (in capsules) or magnesium stearate (a flow agent).

2. Recognizing Quality with Third-Party Certifications

Many supplements are unregulated and may not meet the claims on their labels. Third-party certifications are a reliable way to ensure quality, potency, and safety.

Important Certifications
- US Pharmacopeia (USP): Confirms that the product contains the nutrients listed at the stated potency and is free from harmful contaminants.
- NSF International: Certifies that the product meets strict standards for quality, safety, and manufacturing.
- ConsumerLab: Independently tests supplements for label accuracy and ingredient safety.
- Informed-Sport/Informed-Choice: Tests for banned substances, especially useful for athletes.
- Non-GMO Verified: Ensures that the product does not contain genetically modified organisms.

How to Verify Certifications
Look for certification logos on the packaging.

Cross-check the brand or product on the certifying organization's website.

3. Avoiding Counterfeit and Low-Quality Products

Counterfeit supplements can contain incorrect doses, harmful additives, or even no active ingredients. To avoid these risks, follow these guidelines:

Red Flags of Low-Quality Products
- Too Good to Be True Claims: Beware of promises like "instant results" or "cures all diseases."
- Vague Ingredients: Look out for terms like "proprietary blend" without specific details on quantities.
- No Third-Party Testing: Lack of certifications suggests a product may not meet quality standards.
- Non-Transparent Companies: Avoid brands that don't disclose their manufacturing practices or ingredient sources.

Tips for Buying Safely
- Stick to Trusted Retailers: Buy from reputable stores, pharmacies, or the supplement manufacturer's official website.
- Inspect Packaging: Look for sealed containers, clear labeling, and proper expiration dates.
- Check Batch Numbers: Quality brands often include batch numbers for traceability.

4. Choosing the Right Type of Supplement

Not all forms of vitamins are created equal. Depending on your needs and preferences, certain types may work better for you.

Forms of Supplements
- Capsules: Easy to swallow and often free from unnecessary additives.
- Tablets: Compact and cost-effective but may include binders or coatings.
- Powders: Useful for larger doses (e.g., protein powders with added vitamins).

- Chewables: Ideal for children or adults who dislike swallowing pills.
- Liquid Drops: Fast absorption, especially for fat-soluble vitamins like Vitamin D.

Bioavailability Matters

Some forms of vitamins are more readily absorbed than others.

Example: Methylcobalamin (Vitamin B12) is more bioavailable than cyanocobalamin.

Example: Magnesium citrate is better absorbed than magnesium oxide.

5. Tailoring Supplements to Your Needs

Before buying a supplement, consider your individual health profile and lifestyle.

Key Questions to Ask

✓*Do I Really Need This Supplement?*

If you have a balanced diet, you may not need a multivitamin.

For specific deficiencies (e.g., iron or Vitamin D), supplementation may be necessary.

✓*What Are My Lifestyle Factors?*

Vegetarians/Vegans: Look for B12, iron, and Omega-3 supplements.

Active Individuals: May require extra B-complex vitamins and magnesium.

✓*Do I Have Specific Health Conditions?*

Pregnant women should prioritize folic acid, iron, and calcium.

Seniors may need B12, D3, and calcium due to decreased absorption.

6. Understanding Dosage and Safety

Avoid Megadosing

More is not always better. Taking excessive doses of vitamins can lead to toxicity, particularly with fat-soluble vitamins like A, D, E, and K.

Example: The tolerable upper intake level (UL) for Vitamin D is 4,000 IU per day for adults. Excess can cause hypercalcemia.

Follow Recommended Guidelines

Stick to the RDA or a dosage recommended by your healthcare provider.

Use caution with high-potency supplements unless prescribed for a deficiency.

7. Trends to Watch in the Supplement Industry

The supplement market is evolving, with new innovations designed to improve efficacy and convenience.

- Sustainably Sourced Products: Growing demand for eco-friendly supplements is driving innovations in algae-based Omega-3 and plant-based Vitamin D.
- Advanced Delivery Systems: Liposomal and nano-emulsion technologies improve bioavailability.

Conclusion: An Informed Approach to Supplements

Choosing the right vitamin supplement requires a balance of knowledge, discernment, and self-awareness. By understanding how to read labels, verifying certifications, and assessing your personal needs, you can confidently navigate the world of supplements.

CHAPTER 5:

VITAMINS AND DISEASE PREVENTION – THE GUARDIANS OF LONG–TERM HEALTH

Vitamins play a pivotal role in maintaining overall health, but their influence extends far beyond day-to-day bodily functions. As science advances, researchers have uncovered the ways in which vitamins contribute to preventing chronic diseases like heart disease, diabetes, and even cancer.

This chapter explores the profound role vitamins play in combating disease, delves into the science of antioxidants, and addresses controversies surrounding their effectiveness in boosting immunity and preventing illnesses like the common cold.

The Role of Vitamins in Preventing Chronic Diseases

1. Heart Disease

Heart disease, including conditions like coronary artery disease and hypertension, is one of the leading causes of death worldwide. Vitamins can play a preventative role by addressing factors like inflammation, cholesterol levels, and oxidative stress.

✦Vitamin D:

Helps regulate blood pressure by improving calcium metabolism and reducing arterial stiffness. Studies suggest that individuals with sufficient Vitamin D levels have a lower risk of developing cardiovascular disease.

Scientific Insight: A 2018 meta-analysis in the journal Circulation highlighted an inverse relationship between Vitamin D levels and hypertension.

✦Vitamin B-complex (B6, B9, B12):

These vitamins help reduce homocysteine levels, an amino acid linked to heart disease when present in high amounts. Folic acid

(Vitamin B9) is particularly effective in preventing arterial damage. Scientific Insight: Research published in The Lancet demonstrated that folic acid supplementation reduces stroke risk, especially in populations with low dietary folate intake.

✦Vitamin E:

An antioxidant that prevents oxidative damage to LDL cholesterol, reducing plaque buildup in arteries. However, large-scale studies have yielded mixed results on its effectiveness in reducing heart disease risk.

2. Diabetes

Vitamins may help prevent or manage Type 2 diabetes by improving insulin sensitivity and reducing complications associated with the disease.

✦Vitamin D:

Plays a critical role in insulin secretion and glucose metabolism. Deficiency has been linked to an increased risk of Type 2 diabetes. Scientific Insight: A study in Diabetes Care (2011) found that higher levels of Vitamin D were associated with a lower risk of developing diabetes.

✦Vitamin C:

Helps reduce oxidative stress, which is a major contributor to diabetes complications like neuropathy and kidney damage. Scientific Insight: Antioxidant therapy, including Vitamin C, has been shown to improve vascular function in diabetics, as reported in the journal Free Radical Biology and Medicine.

✦Vitamin B1 (Thiamine):

Deficiency in thiamine is common in diabetics and can worsen complications like cardiovascular issues. Supplements may help protect against kidney and nerve damage.

3. Cancer

The relationship between vitamins and cancer prevention is

complex, with certain vitamins showing promise in reducing risk while others are under scrutiny.

✦Vitamin D:
Sufficient Vitamin D levels are associated with a reduced risk of colon, breast, and prostate cancers. The vitamin helps regulate cell growth and apoptosis (programmed cell death), which are crucial in preventing cancer development.
Scientific Insight: A 2020 study in JAMA Network Open showed that Vitamin D supplementation lowered the risk of advanced cancer in individuals with normal BMI.

✦Vitamin C:
Acts as an antioxidant, protecting cells from DNA damage caused by free radicals. Intravenous Vitamin C has been explored as a potential complementary treatment for cancer, though its efficacy remains controversial.

✦Vitamin A and Beta-Carotene:
These nutrients support cell differentiation and immune function, potentially lowering cancer risk. However, excessive supplementation, particularly of beta-carotene, has been linked to increased lung cancer risk in smokers.

Vitamins as Antioxidants and Their Role in Combating Oxidative Stress

Oxidative stress occurs when there is an imbalance between free radicals (unstable molecules) and antioxidants in the body. Over time, oxidative stress can damage cells, contributing to aging and the development of chronic diseases like cancer, Alzheimer's, and cardiovascular conditions.

Key Antioxidant Vitamins
- Vitamin C: Neutralizes free radicals and regenerates other antioxidants like Vitamin E.
- Vitamin E: Protects cell membranes from oxidative damage.

- Vitamin A: Supports immune function and protects DNA from oxidative damage.

Scientific Evidence

A 2016 study in Nutrients highlighted how a diet rich in antioxidant vitamins reduced markers of oxidative stress and inflammation in individuals with chronic diseases.

Research suggests that antioxidant-rich diets, such as the Mediterranean diet, are linked to lower incidences of heart disease and certain cancers.

However, excessive reliance on supplements rather than whole foods can lead to diminished benefits, as the body prefers antioxidants in their natural, food-based form.

Controversies: Are Vitamins Effective in Boosting Immunity or Preventing Colds?

√ The Case for Vitamin C
Vitamin C has long been promoted as a go-to remedy for colds, but scientific evidence paints a mixed picture.
- Supporting Evidence: Regular Vitamin C supplementation has been shown to reduce the duration and severity of colds, especially in individuals under physical stress (e.g., athletes).
- Skepticism: For the general population, Vitamin C does not prevent colds but may offer minor benefits once symptoms appear.

√ The Role of Vitamin D in Immunity
Vitamin D plays a crucial role in modulating the immune system. Deficiency has been linked to increased susceptibility to respiratory infections, including influenza.
- Scientific Insight: A 2017 meta-analysis in BMJ found that Vitamin D supplementation significantly reduced the risk of acute respiratory infections, particularly in individuals with severe deficiencies.

√ Zinc and Immunity

Though not a vitamin, zinc is often included in immune-boosting supplements. It has been shown to reduce the duration of colds when taken within 24 hours of symptom onset.

The Controversy of Multivitamins

- Proponents: Multivitamins can help fill nutrient gaps and potentially strengthen the immune system, particularly in individuals with deficiencies.
- Critics: Studies, including one in Annals of Internal Medicine (2013), suggest that multivitamins provide little benefit for preventing chronic diseases or enhancing immunity in well-nourished individuals.

Balancing Expectations and Reality

While vitamins are vital for overall health, they are not magic bullets. Over-reliance on supplements can lead to complacency in other areas of health, such as diet, exercise, and sleep.

What Does the Evidence Say?

Whole foods remain the best source of vitamins, as they provide synergistic benefits that isolated supplements cannot replicate.

Supplements should be used as an adjunct, not a replacement, for a balanced diet.

Conclusion

The role of vitamins in preventing chronic diseases and boosting immunity is supported by scientific evidence, but it comes with caveats. While some vitamins show clear benefits in specific contexts, others offer limited or mixed results. The key lies in understanding your unique needs, adopting a nutrient-rich diet, and using supplements judiciously under medical guidance.

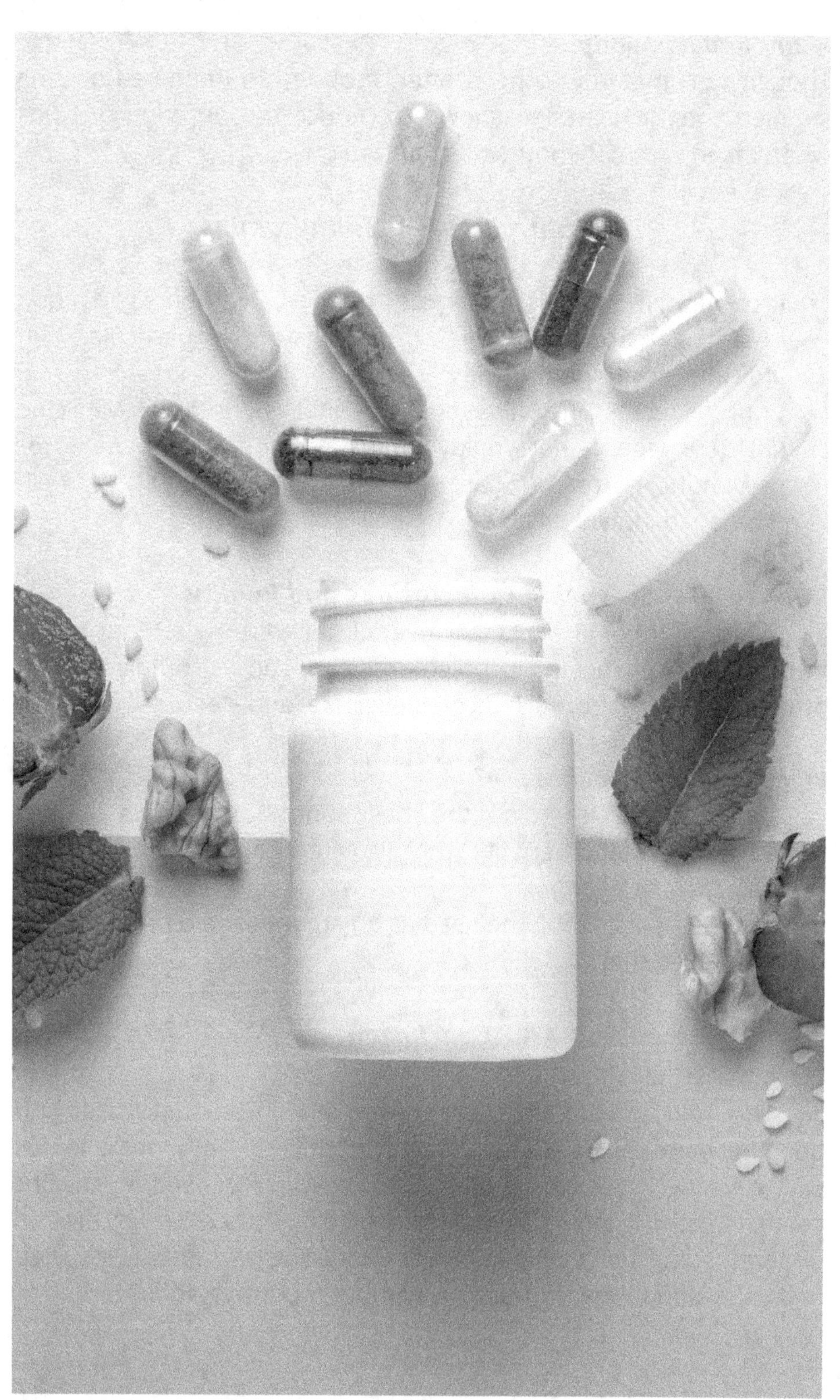

CHAPTER 6:

PERSONALIZED VITAMIN NEEDS – ONE SIZE DOESN'T FIT ALL

When it comes to vitamins, a one-size-fits-all approach simply doesn't work. Each person's body is unique, influenced by genetics, lifestyle, health conditions, and even the environment. As nutritional science advances, so does our understanding of personalized vitamin needs.

This chapter explores the factors shaping individual vitamin requirements, how modern technology is revolutionizing supplementation, and real-world examples of personalized approaches to nutrition.

Factors That Influence Vitamin Needs

1. Genetics: The Blueprint of Nutrition

Genetics plays a critical role in how our bodies process and utilize vitamins. Variations in certain genes can affect:

- Absorption: Some individuals may have difficulty absorbing specific vitamins, like Vitamin B12 or Vitamin D.
- Metabolism: Genetic differences can influence how efficiently vitamins are converted into their active forms (e.g., converting beta-carotene into Vitamin A).
- Requirements: Variations in the MTHFR gene can increase the need for folate (Vitamin B9), impacting energy production and DNA repair.

Example:
People with a genetic predisposition to celiac disease may struggle to absorb fat-soluble vitamins (A, D, E, K) due to intestinal damage.

2. Age and Life Stages

Vitamin needs fluctuate throughout life.

- Infancy and Childhood: Rapid growth demands higher levels of

51

Vitamins A, D, and calcium for bone development.

- Pregnancy and Lactation: Nutrient requirements increase to support fetal development, with folic acid (B9) and iron being critical.
- Older Adults: Aging reduces nutrient absorption, particularly Vitamin B12 and Vitamin D, increasing the risk of deficiencies.

Example:
Postmenopausal women are often prescribed calcium and Vitamin D supplements to prevent osteoporosis.

3. Gender and Hormonal Differences

Men and women have distinct nutritional needs due to hormonal and physiological differences.

- Women: Require more iron during menstruation and pregnancy.
- Men: May need higher doses of certain antioxidants like Vitamin C and E due to greater oxidative stress from higher muscle mass.

Example:
Women with polycystic ovary syndrome (PCOS) may benefit from Vitamin D and inositol supplements to regulate hormones and improve fertility.

4. Health Conditions and Medications

Chronic illnesses and certain medications can alter vitamin requirements.

- Diabetes: Increases the need for antioxidants like Vitamin C and E to combat oxidative stress.
- Kidney Disease: Can lead to deficiencies in Vitamin D and B-complex vitamins.
- Medications: Long-term use of antacids can reduce Vitamin B12 absorption, while diuretics may deplete magnesium and potassium.

5. Lifestyle and Environmental Factors

- Dietary Choices: Vegans may require supplementation of B12, iron, and Omega-3 fatty acids.

- Activity Levels: Athletes have higher needs for B-complex vitamins to support energy metabolism.
- Environment: People living in northern climates often need more Vitamin D due to limited sunlight exposure.

Conclusion: A New Era of Vitamin Wellness

Personalized vitamin regimens represent the next frontier in preventive health care. By understanding the unique factors influencing nutrient needs and leveraging modern technology, individuals can optimize their health like never before. The future of vitamins lies not in a single multivitamin pill for everyone, but in tailored solutions designed for the individual.

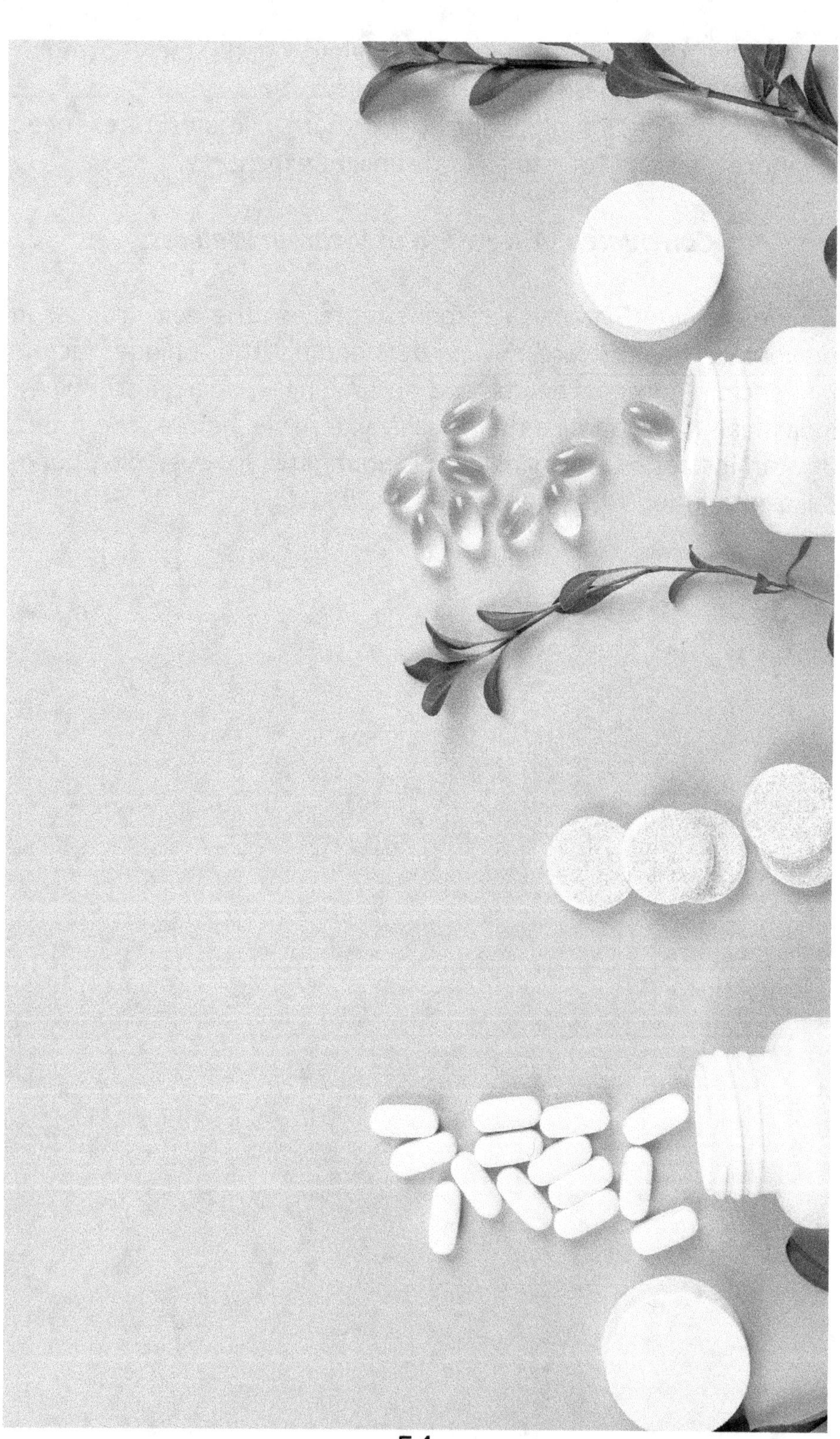

<h1 style="text-align:center">CHAPTER 7:</h1>

<h1 style="text-align:center">NATURAL VERSUS SYNTHETIC VITAMINS – WHAT'S THE DIFFERENCE?</h1>

When walking through the supplement aisle or browsing online, you've likely seen claims like "all-natural" or "lab-tested synthetic" vitamins. But what do these terms actually mean? Are natural vitamins better than synthetic ones? How can you ensure that the supplements you're buying are high-quality and effective?

In this chapter, we'll explore the differences between natural and synthetic vitamins, their effectiveness, and how to make informed choices.

Natural vs. Synthetic Vitamins: The Basics

What Are Natural Vitamins?

Natural vitamins are derived from whole food sources, such as fruits, vegetables, and animal products. They are extracted or concentrated without significant chemical alterations.
Example: Vitamin C from acerola cherries or citrus fruits.

Key Feature: Accompanied by other beneficial nutrients like phytonutrients, fiber, and enzymes that may enhance their absorption and effectiveness.

What Are Synthetic Vitamins?

Synthetic vitamins are made in laboratories using chemical processes. They are designed to mimic the molecular structure of vitamins found in nature.
Example: Ascorbic acid (Vitamin C) produced from glucose in a lab.

Key Feature: Isolated and purified, often free from other nutrients naturally found in food.

Comparing Effectiveness and Bioavailability

1. Bioavailability: How Well Are They Absorbed?

Bioavailability refers to how easily a vitamin is absorbed and utilized by the body.

- Natural Vitamins: Often more bioavailable because they come with co-factors (e.g., Vitamin C from oranges comes with flavonoids that enhance absorption).
- Synthetic Vitamins: Some forms are equally bioavailable (e.g., synthetic ascorbic acid is nearly identical to natural Vitamin C), but others may have reduced effectiveness.

Example:

Synthetic Vitamin E (dl-alpha-tocopherol) is less bioavailable than natural Vitamin E (d-alpha-tocopherol), meaning the body absorbs and uses less of the synthetic version.

2. Composition: The Whole Versus the Isolated

- Natural Vitamins: Provide additional nutrients like antioxidants, fiber, and enzymes that synergize with the vitamin.
- Synthetic Vitamins: Offer the isolated compound, which may be less effective without complementary nutrients.

Example:

Natural Vitamin C from citrus fruits includes bioflavonoids, which may enhance its antioxidant effects compared to isolated ascorbic acid.

3. Effectiveness: Does It Work the Same?

While some synthetic vitamins perform well, others may fall short:

√ Better as Natural:

- Vitamin E: The natural form is more effective in reducing oxidative stress.
- Beta-Carotene (a precursor to Vitamin A): Synthetic forms have been linked to increased lung cancer risk in smokers, while natural sources are safer.

√ Equally Effective:

- Vitamin D: Both natural (from lanolin or fish liver oil) and synthetic (ergocalciferol or cholecalciferol) forms are effective when properly dosed.

- Vitamin B12: Synthetic cyanocobalamin and natural methylcobalamin are both effective, though the latter is slightly preferred for those with certain health conditions.

Pros and Cons of Each

✦Natural Vitamins

Pros:
- Often more bioavailable.
- Accompanied by co-factors for better absorption.
- Derived from whole foods, making them suitable for clean-label enthusiasts.

Cons:
- More expensive due to complex extraction processes.
- May contain allergens or contaminants if poorly sourced.
- Potency can vary depending on the source and processing.

✦Synthetic Vitamins

Pros:
- Cost-effective and widely available.
- Consistent potency and purity.
- Essential for fortifying foods (e.g., folic acid in flour to prevent neural tube defects).

Cons:
- May lack co-factors for optimal absorption.
- Some forms are less bioavailable.
- Over-reliance can lead to imbalances or deficiencies in other nutrients.

How to Identify High-Quality Supplements

With so many options on the market, identifying high-quality vitamins requires careful attention to labels, sourcing, and certifications.

1. Look for Trusted Certifications

Certifications indicate that a supplement has been independently tested for quality and safety.
- US Pharmacopeia (USP): Ensures accurate labeling, purity, and potency.

- NSF International: Verifies good manufacturing practices (GMP) and contaminant-free products.
- ConsumerLab: Tests for quality and accurate labeling.

2. Check the Ingredient List
- Natural Sources: Look for terms like "from acerola cherries," "sourced from algae," or "derived from fish oil."
- Synthetic Forms: Common terms include "ascorbic acid" (Vitamin C), "dl-alpha-tocopherol" (Vitamin E), or "cyanocobalamin" (Vitamin B12).
- Avoid Unnecessary Additives: Watch out for artificial colors, flavors, or fillers.

3. Research the Brand
Look for transparency about sourcing and manufacturing processes.

Read reviews or consult independent testing organizations.

4. Be Wary of Bold Claims
Supplements that claim to "cure diseases," "boost energy instantly," or "detoxify your body" are likely marketing gimmicks. Vitamins are essential nutrients, not miracle drugs.

5. Consider Third-Party Testing
Independent testing labs like Labdoor provide unbiased evaluations of supplement quality, ranking products based on safety, efficacy, and value.

Making the Right Choice for You

The decision between natural and synthetic vitamins depends on your individual needs, budget, and health goals:

✓If You Prefer Whole Foods: Opt for natural vitamins from reputable brands that extract nutrients from food sources.

✓If You Need Targeted Support: Synthetic vitamins can provide precise doses and specific formulations (e.g., prenatal vitamins or Vitamin D3 supplements).

✔If You Have Allergies or Sensitivities: Synthetic vitamins may be a better choice because they are free from common allergens found in food-based supplements.

Conclusion: A Balanced Perspective

Natural and synthetic vitamins each have their place in health and nutrition. Natural vitamins, with their accompanying co-factors, may offer enhanced bioavailability and effectiveness in certain cases, while synthetic vitamins provide consistency and accessibility.

Ultimately, the best vitamin is the one that meets your unique needs, is sourced responsibly, and aligns with your health goals. By understanding the differences and choosing high-quality supplements, you can take a thoughtful and informed approach to maintaining your health.

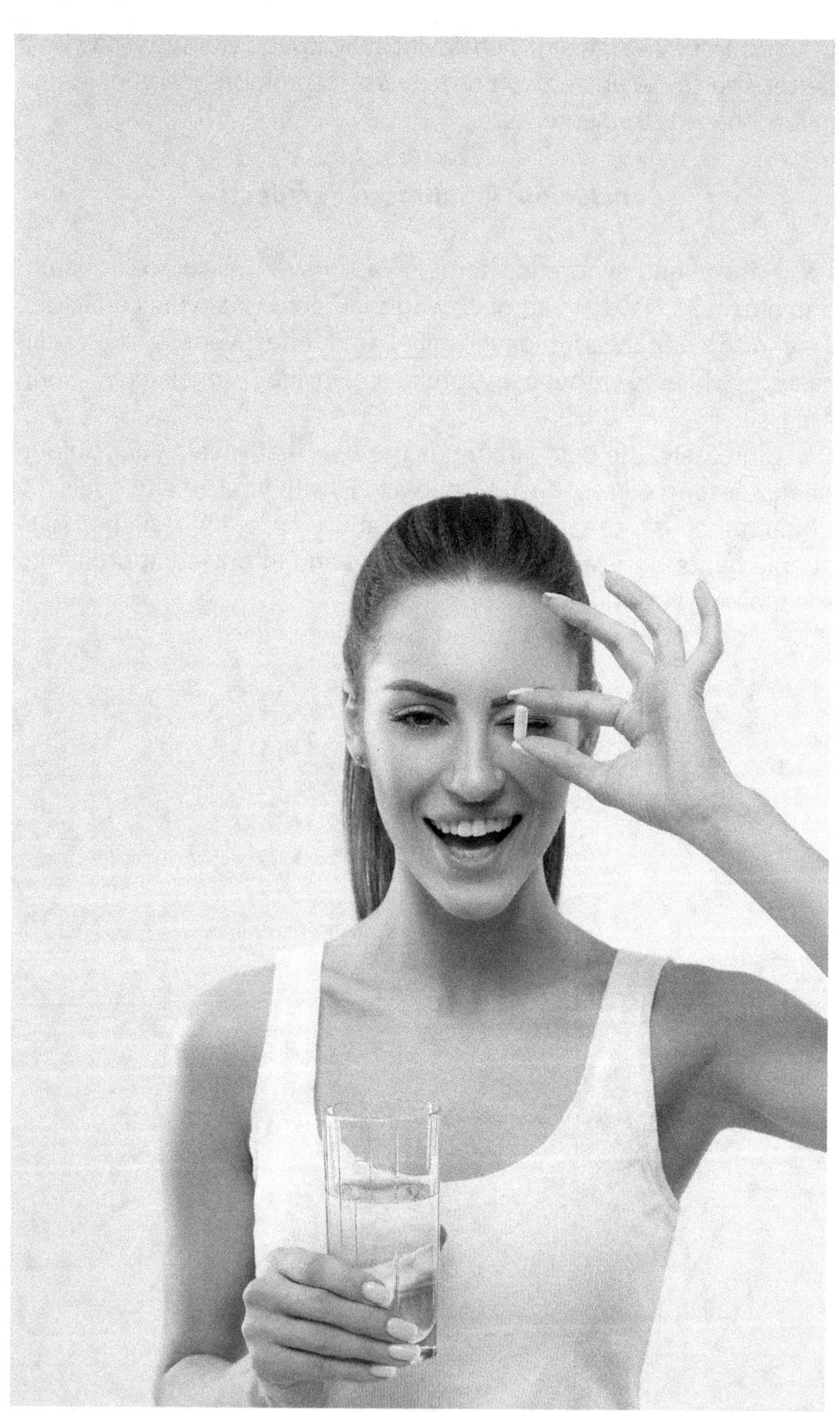

CHAPTER 8:

VITAMINS AND BEAUTY – THE SECRET TO RADIANT SKIN, HAIR, AND NAILS

Beauty isn't just skin-deep—it starts with the nutrients your body absorbs. Vitamins play a vital role in maintaining healthy, glowing skin, lustrous hair, and strong nails.

This chapter explores the science behind beauty-enhancing vitamins, identifies common deficiencies that lead to aesthetic issues, and provides fun DIY recipes for creating vitamin-infused beauty treatments.

The Beauty Vitamins: Their Role in Skin, Hair, and Nail Health

1. Vitamin A: The Skin Protector
Vitamin A is essential for skin renewal, helping to maintain a smooth and youthful appearance.

How It Helps:
- Promotes cell turnover, reducing wrinkles and fine lines.
- Fights acne by preventing clogged pores.
- Strengthens the skin barrier, keeping it hydrated and resilient.

Sources: Sweet potatoes, carrots, spinach, eggs, and fortified milk.

Deficiency Signs: Dry, flaky skin, rough patches, and delayed wound healing.

Beauty Tip: Retinol, a derivative of Vitamin A, is widely used in anti-aging and acne treatments.

2. Vitamin E: The Skin and Hair Healer

Vitamin E is a powerful antioxidant that protects cells from oxidative damage.

How It Helps:
- Prevents skin damage caused by UV rays.
- Promotes scalp health and hair growth.
- Hydrates skin and reduces the appearance of scars.

Sources: Almonds, sunflower seeds, spinach, and avocado.

Deficiency Signs: Dry skin, hair thinning, and poor wound healing.

Beauty Tip: Combine Vitamin E oil with your favorite moisturizer for added hydration and scar reduction.

3. Vitamin C: The Glow Booster

Vitamin C is a superstar for achieving radiant, youthful skin.

How It Helps:
- Stimulates collagen production, improving skin elasticity.
- Brightens the skin by reducing dark spots and hyperpigmentation.
- Protects against free radical damage from pollution and sunlight.

Sources: Oranges, strawberries, bell peppers, and kiwis.

Deficiency Signs: Dull skin, slow wound healing, and weakened nails.

Beauty Tip: Incorporate Vitamin C serums into your skincare routine to brighten and firm your skin.

4. Biotin (Vitamin B7): The Hair and Nail Strengthener

Biotin is famous for its ability to promote strong, healthy hair and nails.

How It Helps:
- Strengthens keratin, the protein that forms hair, skin, and nails.
- Prevents hair thinning and promotes growth.
- Reduces brittleness in nails.

Sources: Eggs, nuts, seeds, and whole grains.

Deficiency Signs: Hair loss, brittle nails, and skin rashes.

Beauty Tip: Consider a biotin supplement if you notice persistent hair or nail brittleness, but consult your doctor first.

5. Other Key Vitamins for Beauty

✦***Vitamin D:*** Essential for hair follicle health; deficiency can lead to hair thinning.
Sources: Sunlight, fatty fish, fortified dairy.

✦***Vitamin B-complex:*** Supports skin hydration, reduces redness, and enhances hair growth.
Sources: Leafy greens, whole grains, and lean meats.

✦***Vitamin K:*** Reduces under-eye circles and improves skin elasticity.
Sources: Kale, spinach, broccoli, and fermented foods.

Common Deficiencies and Their Beauty Impact

1. Skin Issues
- Dry Skin: Linked to deficiencies in Vitamin A, E, and essential fatty acids.
- Acne and Redness: Low levels of Vitamin A and zinc may exacerbate inflammation.
- Dull Complexion: Vitamin C deficiency reduces collagen production, causing sagging and uneven skin tone.

2. Hair Problems
- Hair Thinning: Commonly caused by low Vitamin D, biotin, or iron levels.

- Brittle Hair: Deficiency in Vitamin E or essential fatty acids weakens hair strands.

3. Nail Concerns

- Brittle Nails: Often linked to biotin deficiency.
- Ridges in Nails: A sign of low iron, Vitamin B12, or zinc.

DIY RECIPES FOR VITAMIN-INFUSED BEAUTY TREATMENTS

1. Vitamin C Brightening Serum

INGREDIENTS:

1 teaspoon Vitamin C powder (ascorbic acid).
2 tablespoons distilled water.
1 teaspoon aloe vera gel.
5 drops Vitamin E oil (optional).

INSTRUCTIONS:

- Dissolve Vitamin C powder in distilled water.
- Mix in aloe vera gel and Vitamin E oil.
- Store in a dark glass bottle and refrigerate.
- Apply a few drops to your face in the morning before moisturizer.
- Benefits: Brightens skin, reduces dark spots, and boosts collagen.

2. Biotin Hair Growth Mask

INGREDIENTS:

1 ripe avocado.
1 egg yolk (rich in biotin).
1 tablespoon coconut oil.

- Mash the avocado and mix with egg yolk.
- Add coconut oil and blend until smooth.
- Apply to damp hair, focusing on the scalp.
- Leave for 20-30 minutes, then rinse with shampoo.
- Benefits: Deeply nourishes the scalp and strengthens hair strands.

3. *Vitamin E Nail Strengthening Oil*

INGREDIENTS:

2 tablespoons olive oil.
1 teaspoon Vitamin E oil.
5 drops lavender essential oil (optional).

INSTRUCTIONS:

- Mix all ingredients in a small bottle.
- Massage a few drops into your nails and cuticles daily.
- Benefits: Prevents brittleness and promotes nail growth.

4. *Vitamin A Hydrating Face Mask*

INGREDIENTS:

1 small carrot, boiled and mashed.
1 tablespoon honey.
1 teaspoon plain yogurt.

INSTRUCTIONS:

- Blend all ingredients until smooth.

- Apply to your face and leave for 15-20 minutes.
- Rinse with warm water.
- Benefits: Hydrates skin, promotes cell turnover, and reduces fine lines.

How to Incorporate Beauty Vitamins into Your Routine

- Eat a Balanced Diet: Focus on whole foods rich in beauty vitamins.
- Supplement Wisely: Use supplements to address specific deficiencies, but consult a healthcare provider first.
- Topical Applications: Serums and creams infused with vitamins can target specific concerns like wrinkles or dullness.
- Stay Consistent: Results from vitamins often take weeks or months to show, so be patient.

Conclusion: Beauty from the Inside Out

Vitamins are the unsung heroes of beauty, working beneath the surface to keep your skin radiant, your hair shiny, and your nails strong. By nourishing your body with the right nutrients and incorporating vitamin-rich foods and treatments into your routine, you can unlock a natural, glowing beauty that reflects true health.

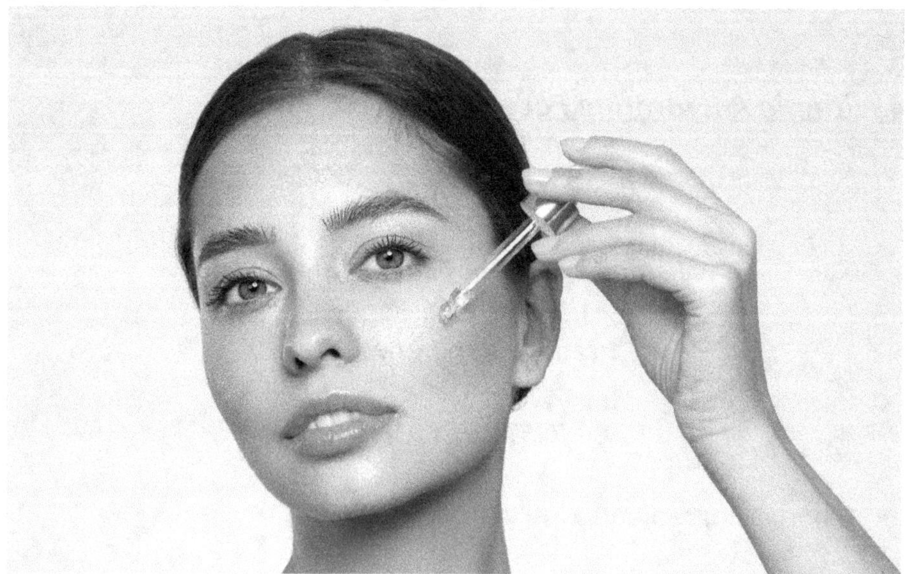

CONCLUSION:

EMBRACING THE POWER OF VITAMINS

As we conclude this journey through the vibrant world of vitamins, one thing becomes abundantly clear: these tiny yet mighty nutrients hold the keys to a healthier, more fulfilling life. From their essential role in maintaining physical and mental well-being to their contributions to beauty, vitality, and disease prevention, vitamins are indispensable allies in our pursuit of optimal health.

A Holistic Approach to Health

The knowledge you've gained from this book is not just about understanding vitamins—it's about embracing a holistic approach to your well-being. Health isn't found in a single supplement or a one-time effort; it's a lifelong commitment to nourishing your body, mind, and spirit. By integrating vitamin-rich foods, making informed choices about supplements, and listening to your body's unique needs, you can create a foundation for vitality that lasts a lifetime.

Empowered Choices for a Vibrant Life

In an age of endless health trends and conflicting advice, you now have the tools to navigate the world of nutrition with confidence. Whether it's decoding supplement labels, personalizing your vitamin intake, or crafting DIY beauty treatments, your understanding of vitamins empowers you to make choices that truly support your goals and values.

Looking Ahead

The science of vitamins continues to evolve, and with it, our understanding of their potential. As research advances, the connection between nutrition and health will become even clearer, offering new opportunities to harness the power of vitamins in ways we've yet to imagine.

A Final Word

Remember, health is a journey, not a destination. Every meal you eat, every lifestyle choice you make, and every supplement you take is a step toward the vibrant, balanced life you deserve. With the knowledge and insights from this book, you are better equipped to unlock the full potential of your health, beauty, and happiness.

Thank you for embarking on this journey. May the power of vitamins guide you toward a brighter, healthier future!